BLACKWELL'S
UNDERGROUND CLINICAL VIGNETTES

BASIC SCIENCE COLOR ATLAS, STEP 1

BLACKWELL'S
UNDERGROUND CLINICAL VIGNETTES

BASIC SCIENCE COLOR ATLAS, STEP 1

VIKAS BHUSHAN, MD
University of California, San Francisco, Class of 1991
Series Editor, Diagnostic Radiologist

VISHAL PALL, MBBS
Government Medical College, Chandigarh, India, Class of 1996
Series Editor, U. of Texas, Galveston, Resident in Internal Medicine &
Preventive Medicine

TAO LE, MD
University of California, San Francisco, Class of 1996

YI-MENG YEN, MD, PHD
University of California Los Angeles, Resident in Orthopaedic Surgery

SRISHTI GUPTA, MD, MPP
Harvard Medical School, Class of 2003

Blackwell
Publishing

CONTRIBUTORS

Sonal Shah, MD
Ross University, Class of 2000

Aliyah Rahemtullah, MD
Massachusetts General Hospital, Resident in Pathology

FACULTY REVIEWER

Kristina Braaten, MD
Massachusetts General Hospital, Fellow in Surgical Pathology

© 2003 by Blackwell Publishing

Blackwell Publishing, Inc., 350 Main Street,
    Malden, Massachusetts 02148-5018, USA
Blackwell Publishing Ltd, 9600 Garsington Road,
    Oxford OX4 2DQ, UK
Blackwell Science Asia Pty Ltd, 550
    Swanston Street, Carlton South,
    Victoria 3053, Australia

03 04 05 06 5 4 3 2 I

ISBN: 1-4051-0383-3
**Blackwell's Undergeround Clinical Vignettes:
    Basic Science Color Atlas, Step 1**

Acquisitions: Laura DeYoung
Development: Amy Nuttbrock
Production: Lorna Hind and Shawn Girsberger
Cover design: Leslie Haimes
Interior design: Shawn Girsberger
Typesetter: TechBooks, in Pennsylvania
Printed and bound by Capital City Press,
    in Vermont

For further information on Blackwell Publishing,
    visit our website:
    www.blackwellpublishing.com

Notice:
The indications and dosages of all drugs in this book have been recommended in the medical literature and
conform to the practices of the general community. The medications described do not necessarily have specific approval by the Food and Drug Administration for use in the diseases and dosages for which they are
recommended. The package insert for each drug should be consulted for use and dosage as approved by the
FDA. Because standards for usage change, it is advisable to keep abreast of revised recommendations, partic-
ularly those concerning new drugs.

ACKNOWLEDGMENTS

Throughout the production of this book, we have had the support of many friends and colleagues. Special thanks to our support team including Anu Gupta, Andrea Fellows, Anastasia Anderson, Srishti Gupta, Mona Pall, Jonathan Kirsch and Chirag Amin. For prior contributions we thank Gianni Le Nguyen, Tarun Mathur, Alex Grimm, Sonia Santos and Elizabeth Sanders.

We have enjoyed working with a world-class international publishing group at Blackwell Science, including Laura DeYoung, Amy Nuttbrock, Lisa Flanagan, Shawn Girsberger, Lorna Hind and Gordon Tibbitts. For help with securing images for the entire series we also thank Lee Martin, Kristopher Jones, Tina Panizzi and Peter Anderson at the University of Alabama, the Armed Forces Institute of Pathology, and many of our fellow Blackwell Science authors.

For submitting comments, corrections, editing, proofreading, and assistance across all of the vignette titles in all editions, we collectively thank:

Tara Adamovich, Carolyn Alexander, Kris Alden, Henry E. Aryan, Lynman Bacolor, Natalie Barteneva, Dean Bartholomew, Debashish Behera, Sumit Bhatia, Sanjay Bindra, Dave Brinton, Julianne Brown, Alexander Brownie, Tamara Callahan, David Canes, Bryan Casey, Aaron Caughey, Hebert Chen, Jonathan Cheng, Arnold Cheung, Arnold Chin, Simion Chiosea, Yoon Cho, Samuel Chung, Gretchen Conant, Vladimir Coric, Christopher Cosgrove, Ronald Cowan, Karekin R. Cunningham, A. Sean Dalley, Rama Dandamudi, Sunit Das, Ryan Armando Dave, John David, Emmanuel de la Cruz, Robert DeMello, Navneet Dhillon, Sharmila Dissanaike, David Donson, Adolf Etchegaray, Alea Eusebio, Priscilla A. Frase, David Frenz, Kristin Gaumer, Yohannes Gebreegziabher, Anil Gehi, Tony George, L.M. Gotanco, Parul Goyal, Alex Grimm, Rajeev Gupta, Ahmad Halim, Sue Hall, David Hasselbacher, Tamra Heimert, Michelle Higley, Dan Hoit, Eric Jackson, Tim Jackson, Sundar Jayaraman, Pei-Ni Jone, Aarchan Joshi, Rajni K. Jutla, Faiyaz Kapadi, Seth Karp, Aaron S. Kesselheim, Sana Khan, Andrew Pin-wei Ko, Francis Kong, Paul Konitzky, Warren S. Krackov, Benjamin H.S. Lau, Ann LaCasce, Connie Lee, Scott Lee, Guillermo Lehmann, Kevin Leung, Paul Levett, Warren Levinson, Eric Ley, Ken Lin, Pavel Lobanov, J. Mark Maddox, Aram Mardian, Samir Mehta,

Gil Melmed, Joe Messina, Robert Mosca, Michael Murphy, Vivek Nandkarni, Siva Naraynan, Carvell Nguyen, Linh Nguyen, Deanna Nobleza, Craig Nodurft, George Noumi, Darin T. Okuda, Adam L. Palance, Paul Pamphrus, Jinha Park, Sonny Patel, Ricardo Pietrobon, Riva L. Rahl, Aashita Randeria, Rachan Reddy, Beatriu Reig, Marilou Reyes, Jeremy Richmon, Tai Roe, Rick Roller, Rajiv Roy, Diego Ruiz, Anthony Russell, Sanjay Sahgal, Urmimala Sarkar, John Schilling, Isabell Schmitt, Daren Schuhmacher, Sonal Shah, Fadi Abu Shahin, Mae Sheikh-Ali, Edie Shen, Justin Smith, John Stulak, Lillian Su, Julie Sundaram, Rita Suri, Seth Sweetser, Antonio Talayero, Merita Tan, Mark Tanaka, Eric Taylor, Jess Thompson, Indi Trehan, Raymond Turner, Okafo Uchenna, Eric Uyguanco, Richa Varma, John Wages, Alan Wang, Eunice Wang, Andy Weiss, Amy Williams, Brian Yang, Hany Zaky, Ashraf Zaman and David Zipf.

For generously contributing images to the entire *Underground Clinical Vignette* Step 1 series, we collectively thank the staff at Blackwell Science in Oxford, Boston, and Berlin as well as:

- Axford, J. *Medicine.* Osney Mead: Blackwell Science Ltd, 1996. Figures 2.14, 2.15, 2.16, 2.27, 2.28, 2.31, 2.35, 2.36, 2.38, 2.43, 2.65a, 2.65b, 2.65c, 2.103b, 2.105b, 3.20b, 3.21, 8.27, 8.27b, 8.77b, 8.77c, 10.81b, 10.96a, 12.28a, 14.6, 14.16, 14.50.

- Bannister B, Begg N, Gillespie S. *Infectious Disease, 2ⁿᵈ Edition.* Osney Mead: Blackwell Science Ltd, 2000. Figures 2.8, 3.4, 5.28, 18.10, W5.32, W5.6.

- Berg D. *Advanced Clinical Skills and Physical Diagnosis.* Blackwell Science Ltd., 1999. Figures 7.10, 7.12, 7.13, 7.2, 7.3, 7.7, 7.8, 7.9, 8.1, 8.2, 8.4, 8.5, 9.2, 10.2, 11.3, 11.5, 12.6.

- Cuschieri A, Hennessy TPJ, Greenhalgh RM, Rowley DA, Grace PA. *Clinical Surgery.* Osney Mead: Blackwell Science Ltd, 1996. Figures 13.19, 18.22, 18.33.

- Gillespie SH, Bamford K. *Medical Microbiology and Infection at a Glance.* Osney Mead: Blackwell Science Ltd, 2000. Figures 20, 23.

- Ginsberg L. *Lecture Notes on Neurology, 7ᵗʰ Edition.* Osney Mead: Blackwell Science Ltd, 1999. Figures 12.3, 18.3, 18.3b.

- Elliott T, Hastings M, Desselberger U. *Lecture Notes on Medical Microbiology, 3ʳᵈ Edition.* Osney Mead: Blackwell Science Ltd, 1997. Figures 2, 5, 7, 8, 9, 11, 12, 14, 15, 16, 17, 19, 20, 25, 26, 27, 29, 30, 34, 35, 52.

- Mehta AB, Hoffbrand AV. *Haematology at a Glance.* Osney Mead: Blackwell Science Ltd, 2000. Figures 22.1, 22.2, 22.3.

Please let us know if your name has been missed or misspelled and we will be happy to make the update in the next edition.

We were very pleased with the overwhelmingly positive student feedback for the 2nd edition of our *Underground Clinical Vignettes* series. Well over 100,000 copies of the UCV books are in print and have been used by students all over the world.

Over the last two years we have accumulated and incorporated **over a thousand "updates"** and improvements suggested by you, our readers, including:

- many additions of specific boards and wards testable content

- deletions of redundant and overlapping cases

- reordering and reorganization of all cases in both series

- a new master index by case name in each Atlas

- correction of a few factual errors

- diagnosis and treatment updates

- addition of 5–20 new cases in every book

- and the addition of clinical exam photographs within *UCV— Anatomy*

And most important of all, the third edition sets now include two brand new **COLOR ATLAS** supplements, one for each Clinical Vignette series.

- The *UCV–Basic Science Color Atlas* (*Step 1*) includes over 250 color plates, divided into gross pathology, microscopic pathology (histology), hematology, and microbiology (smears).

- The *UCV–Clinical Science Color Atlas* (*Step 2*) has over 125 color plates, including patient images, dermatology, and funduscopy.

Each atlas image is descriptively captioned and linked to its corresponding Step 1 case, Step 2 case, and/or Step 2 MiniCase.

For your convenience, a **Master Case Index** is located in the back of each Atlas.

How Atlas Links Work:

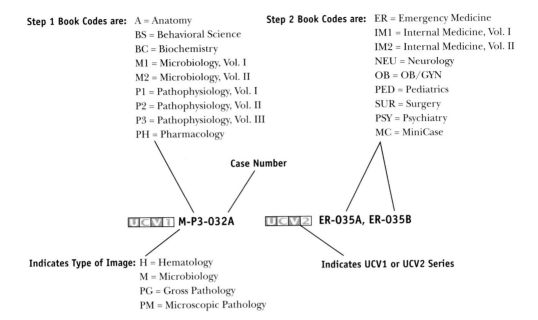

Step 1 Book Codes are:
A = Anatomy
BS = Behavioral Science
BC = Biochemistry
M1 = Microbiology, Vol. I
M2 = Microbiology, Vol. II
P1 = Pathophysiology, Vol. I
P2 = Pathophysiology, Vol. II
P3 = Pathophysiology, Vol. III
PH = Pharmacology

Step 2 Book Codes are:
ER = Emergency Medicine
IM1 = Internal Medicine, Vol. I
IM2 = Internal Medicine, Vol. II
NEU = Neurology
OB = OB/GYN
PED = Pediatrics
SUR = Surgery
PSY = Psychiatry
MC = MiniCase

Case Number

UCV1 M-P3-032A   UCV2 ER-035A, ER-035B

Indicates Type of Image:
H = Hematology
M = Microbiology
PG = Gross Pathology
PM = Microscopic Pathology

Indicates UCV1 or UCV2 Series

- If the Case number (032, 035, etc.) is not followed by a letter, then there is only one image. Otherwise A, B, C, D indicate up to 4 images.

Bold Faced Links: In order to give you access to the largest number of images possible, we have chosen to cross link the Step 1 and 2 series.

- If the link is bold-faced this indicates that the link is direct (i.e., Step 1 Case with the Basic Science Step 1 Atlas link).

- If the link is not bold-faced this indicates that the link is indirect (Step 1 case with Clinical Science Step 2 Atlas link or vice versa).

We have also implemented a few structural changes upon your request:

- Each current and future edition of our popular *First Aid for the USMLE Step 1* (Appleton & Lange/McGraw-Hill) and *First Aid for the USMLE Step 2* (Appleton & Lange/McGraw-Hill) book will be linked to the corresponding UCV case.

- We eliminated UCV → First Aid links as they frequently become out of date, as the *First Aid* books are revised yearly.

- The Color Atlas is also specially designed for quizzing—captions are descriptive and do not give away the case name directly.

We hope the updated UCV series will remain a unique and well-integrated study tool that provides compact clinical correlations to basic science information. They are designed to be easy and fun (comparatively) to read, and helpful for both licensing exams and the wards.

We invite your corrections and suggestions for the fourth edition of these books. For the first submission of each factual correction or new vignette that is selected for inclusion in the fourth edition, you will receive a personal acknowledgment in the revised book. If you submit over 20 high-quality corrections, additions or new vignettes we will also consider **inviting you to become a "Contributor" on the book of your choice**. If you are interested in becoming a potential "Contributor" or "Author" on a future UCV book, or working with our team in developing additional books, please also e-mail us your CV/resume.

We prefer that you submit corrections or suggestions via electronic mail to **UCVteam@yahoo.com**. Please include "Underground Vignettes" as the subject of your message. If you do not have access to e-mail, use the following mailing address: Blackwell Publishing, Attn: UCV Editors, 350 Main Street, Malden, MA 02148, USA.

Vikas Bhushan
Vishal Pall
Tao Le
October 2001

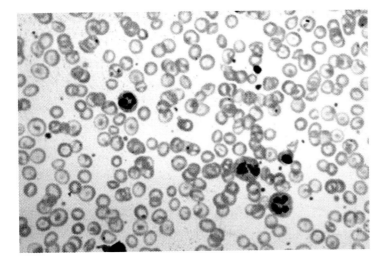

Figure H-BC-077
Ovalocytes with hypersegmented neutrophils.

Text Links:
UCV1 **BC-077**
UCV2 IM1-043

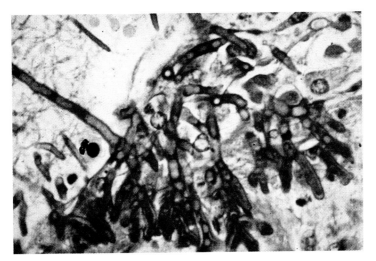

Figure H-M1-046
Giant pronormoblasts.

Text Link:
UCV1 **M1-046**

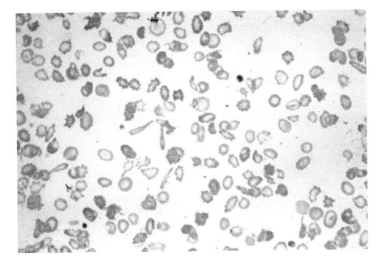

Figure H-M1-049
Fragmented erythro-cytes and a paucity of platelets.

Text Links:
UCV1 **M1-049**
UCV2 MC-124

Figure H-M2-010
Large atypical lymphocyte with enlarged nucleus and abundant cytoplasm.

Text Links:
UCV1 **M2-010**
UCV2 IM2-022

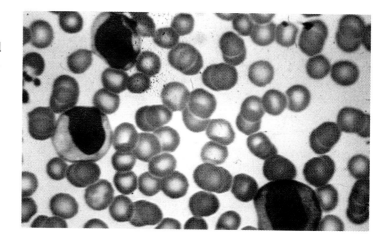

Figure H-M2-014
Amastigote forms of the parasite seen as intracytoplasmic blue particles (LD bodies) in macrophages.

Text Links:
UCV1 **M2-014**
UCV2 MC-178

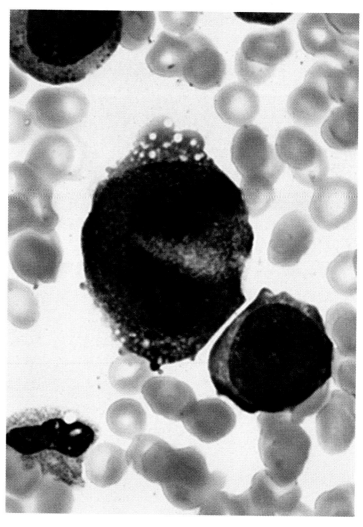

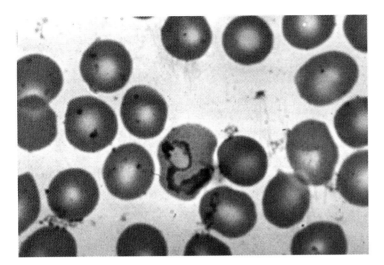

Figure H-M2-022A
Thick smear showing trophozoites.

Text Links:
U C V 1 **M2-022**
U C V 2 MC-181

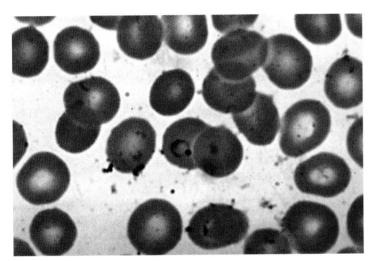

Figure H-M2-022B
Thin smear showing ring-shaped mero-zoites.

Text Links:
U C V 1 **M2-022**
U C V 2 MC-181

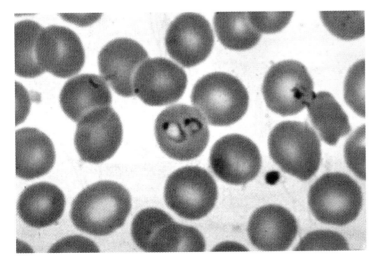

Figure H-M2-022C
Ring-shaped intraery-throcytic merozoites.

Text Links:
U C V 1 **M2-022**
U C V 2 MC-181

Figure H-P1-091
Acanthocytes, macro-
cytes and target cells.

Text Links:
UCV1 **P1-091**
UCV2 IM1-034

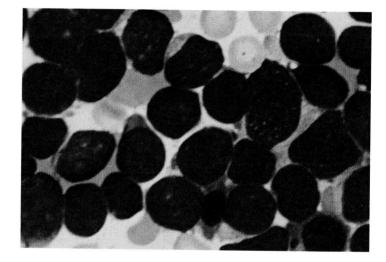

Figure H-P2-013A
Hypercellular bone
marrow aspirate with
immature cells with
large nuclei and scant
basophilic cytoplasm.

Text Links:
UCV1 **P2-013**
UCV2 PED-016

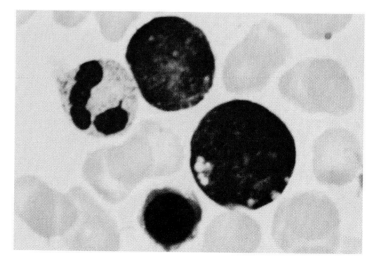

Figure H-P2-013B
Large immature
lymphocyte with
dispersed chromatin
and basophilic cyto-
plasm containing
multiple vacuoles.

Text Links:
UCV1 **P2-013**
UCV2 PED-016

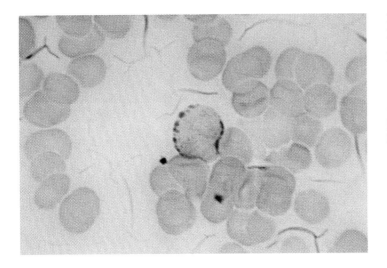

Figure H-P2-013C
Positive periodic acid-Schiff staining in lymphocyte precursor cells.

Text Links:
U C V 1 **P2-013**
U C V 2 PED-016

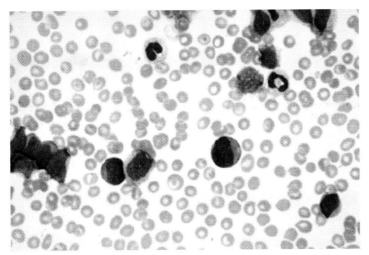

Figure H-P2-014A
Peripheral blood smear demonstrating myeloblasts.

Text Links:
U C V 1 **P2-014**
U C V 2 IM1-041

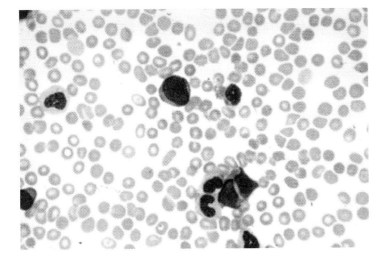

Figure H-P2-014B
Peripheral blood smear demonstrating myeloblasts.

Text Links:
U C V 1 **P2-014**
U C V 2 IM1-041

Figure H-P2-014C
Wright stain of the
bone marrow aspirate
revealing many pleo-
morphic blast cells.

Text Links:
UCV1 **P2-014**
UCV2 IM1-041

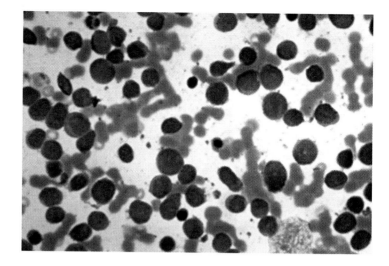

Figure H-P2-014D
Wright stain of the
bone marrow aspirate
revealing many pleo-
morphic blast cells.

Text Links:
UCV1 **P2-014**
UCV2 IM1-041

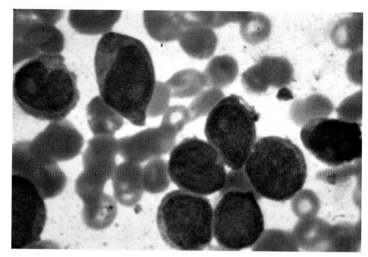

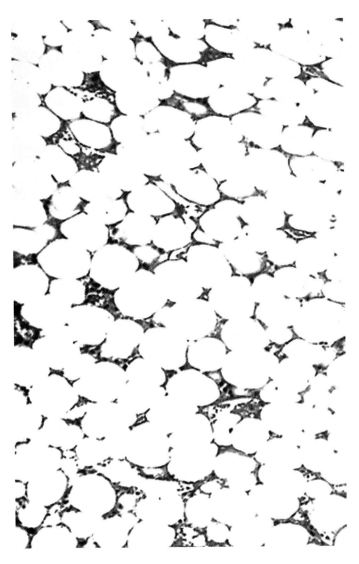

Figure H-P2-015
Extremely hypocellular bone marrow with reticulin fibrosis.

Text Links:
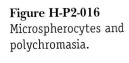 **P2-015**
UCV2 MC-114

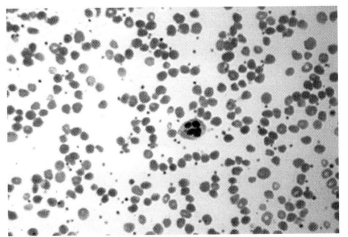

Figure H-P2-016
Microspherocytes and polychromasia.

Text Links:
UCV1 **P2-016**
UCV2 MC-115

Figure H-P2-019
Markedly increased lymphocytes with sparse cytoplasm, round to slightly oval nuclei without evident nucleoli and smudge cells.

Text Links:
UCV1 **P2-019**
UCV2 IM1-045

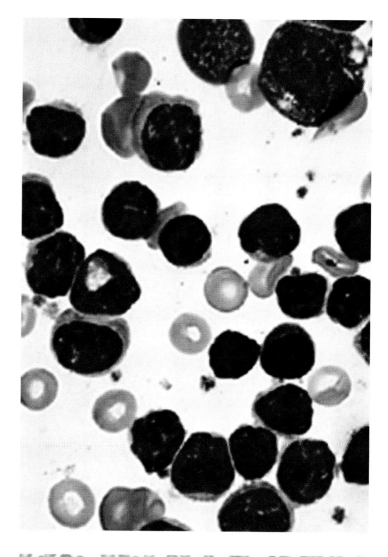

Figure H-P2-020A
Blood smear with leukocytosis and predominant left shift.

Text Links:
UCV1 **P2-020**
UCV2 IM1-046

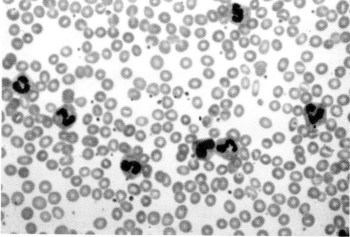

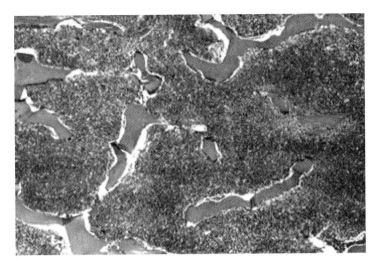

Figure H-P2-020B
Bone marrow biopsy with increased cellularity.

Text Links:
[UCV1] **P2-020**
[UCV2] IM1-046

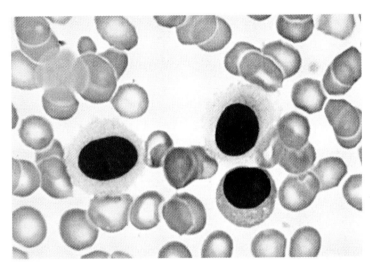

Figure H-P2-024
Blood smear with two "hairy" cells and a plasmacytoid lymphocyte. The cytoplasm of the hairy cells is abundant with "hairy" projections.

Text Links:
[UCV1] **P2-024**
[UCV2] MC-123

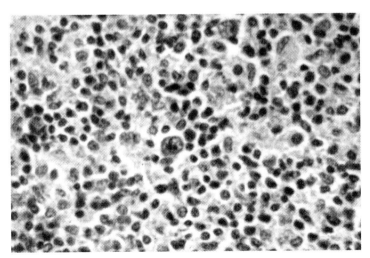

Figure H-P2-029
Lymph node biopsy with central Reed-Sternberg cell surrounded by lymphocytes, neutrophils and eosinophils.

Text Links:
[UCV1] **P2-029**
[UCV2] IM1-049

Figure H-P2-031A
Hypercellular bone
marrow with multinu-
cleated, monomorphic
dysplastic plasma
cells.

Text Links:
⬚U⬚C⬚V⬚1 **P2-031**
⬚U⬚C⬚V⬚2 IM1-050

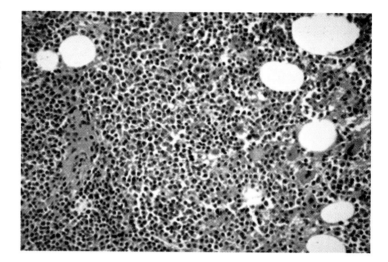

Figure H-P2-031B
Dysplastic plasma
cells.

Text Links:
⬚U⬚C⬚V⬚1 **P2-031**
⬚U⬚C⬚V⬚2 IM1-050

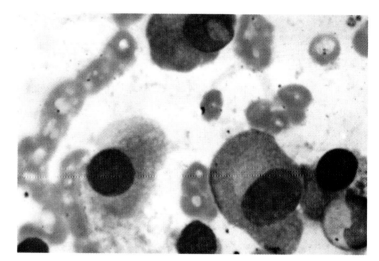

Figure H-P2-032A
Hypocellular fibrotic
bone marrow.

Text Link:
⬚U⬚C⬚V⬚1 **P2-032**

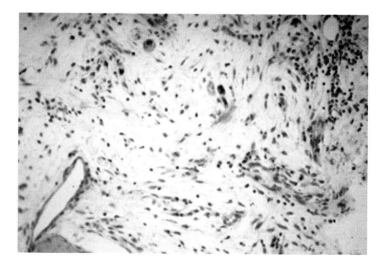

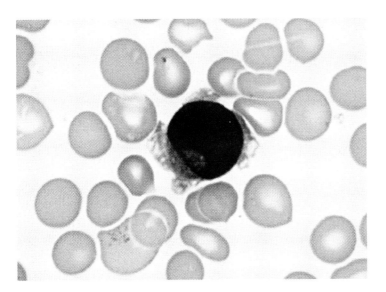

Figure H-P2-032B
Poikilocytosis, aniso-cytosis, nucleated red cells and large platelets.

Text Link:
⬜🅒🆅1 **P2-032**

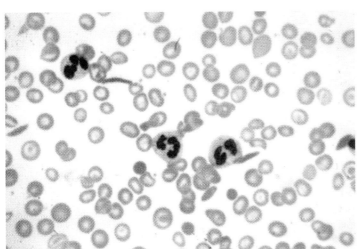

Figure H-P2-036
Sickle cells, anisocy-tosis and target cells.

Text Links:
⬜🅒🆅1 **P2-036**
⬜🅒🆅2 PED-021

Figure M-M1-002
Diffuse lymphocytic infiltration of the myocardium.

Text Links:
UCV1 **M1-002**
UCV2 MC-080

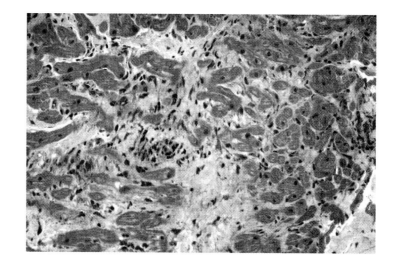

Figure M-M1-012
Short branched hyphae and spores resembling spaghetti and meatballs.

Text Links:
UCV1 **M1-012**
UCV2 MC-148

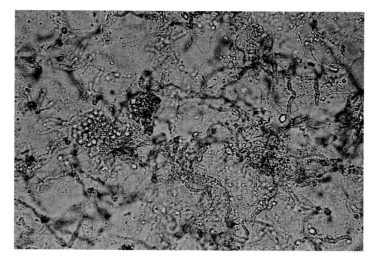

Figure M-M1-026
Long chains of gram-positive cocci.

Text Links:
UCV1 **M1-026**
UCV2 MC-097

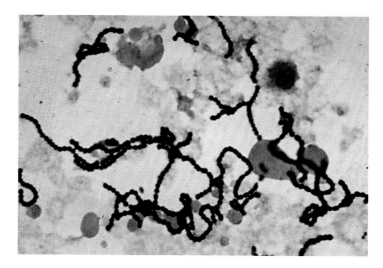

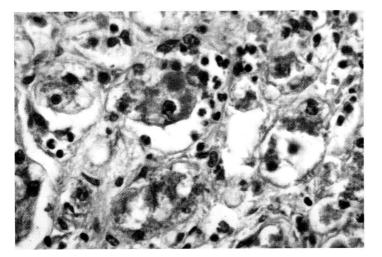

Figure M-M1-030
Hydropic swelling, acidophilic cytoplasmic bodies and necrosis of hepatocytes surrounded by a lymphocytic infiltrate.

Text Link:
U C V 1 M1-030

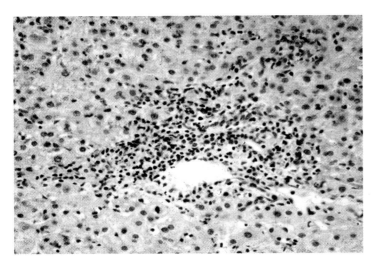

Figure M-M1-031
Lymphoid aggregates in the region of the portal triad.

Text Links:
U C V 1 M1-031
U C V 2 MC-105

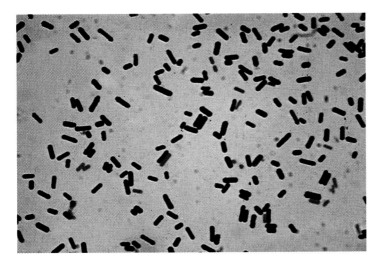

Figure M-M1-033A
Large gram-positive rods.

Text Links:
U C V 1 M1-033
U C V 2 PED-043

Figure M-M1-033B
Zone of hemolysis on
blood agar.

Text Links:
UCV1 **M1-033**
UCV2 PED-043

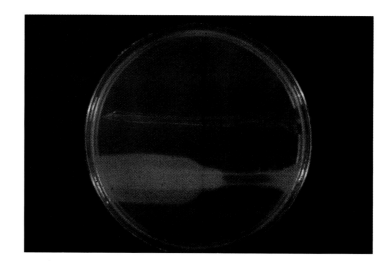

Figure M-M1-035A
Flagellated organism
in gastric mucosa.

Text Links:
UCV1 **M1-035**
UCV2 IM1-038

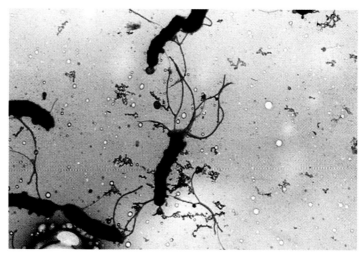

Figure M-M1-035B
Gastric mucosal
biopsy demonstrating
gram-negative spiral
and curved bacilli.

Text Links:
UCV1 **M1-035**
UCV2 IM1-038

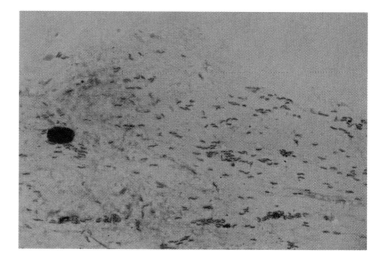

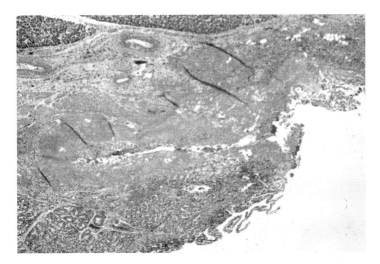

Figure M-M1-035C
Mucosal defect with necrotic base covered with fibrinopurulent exudate.

Text Links:
U C V 1 **M1-035**
U C V 2 IM1-038

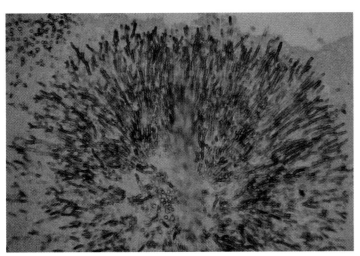

Figure M-M1-050
Gram-variable bacteria in spherical colonies with a branching appearance.

Text Links:
U C V 1 **M1-050**
U C V 2 MC-157

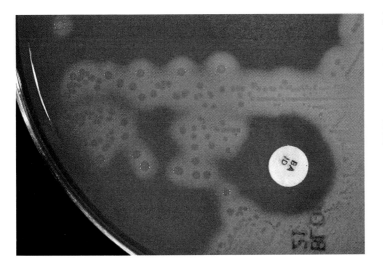

Figure M-M1-052
β-Hemolytic colonies with a zone of inhibition surrounding bacitracin disk.

Text Links:
U C V 1 **M1-052**
U C V 2 PED-025

Figure M-M1-055
Stool specimen show-
ing protozoan cysts.

Text Links:
UCV1 **M1-055**
UCV2 MC-158

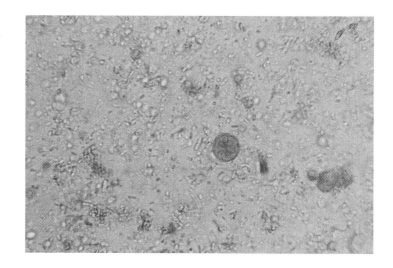

Figure M-M1-059A
Radiating conidia and
parallel filaments with
septae.

Text Links:
UCV1 **M1-059**
UCV2 MC-159

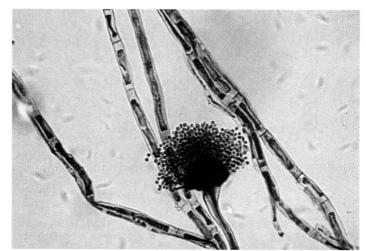

Figure M-M1-059B
Radiating chains of
conidia growing on
Sabouraud's agar.

Text Links:
UCV1 **M1-059**
UCV2 MC-159

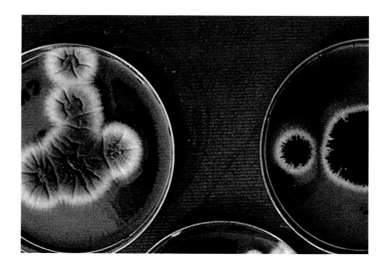

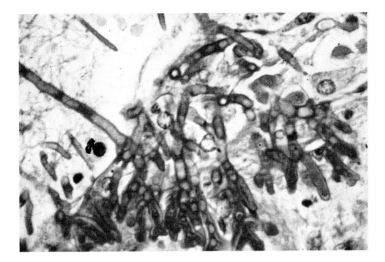

Figure M-M1-059C
Septate, branching hyphae in brain tissue.

Text Links:
U C V 1 **M1-059**
U C V 2 MC-159

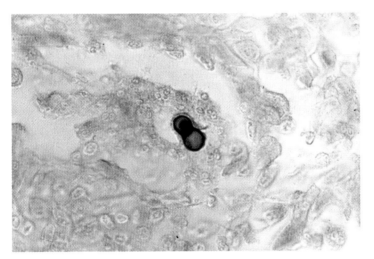

Figure M-M1-065
Biopsy of lung tissue showing an organism with a double con-toured wall and broad based budding.

Text Links:
U C V 1 **M1-065**
U C V 2 MC-161

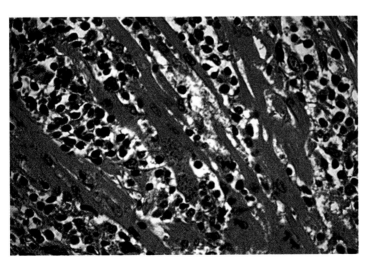

Figure M-M1-071
Parasitic and lympho-cytic infiltration of myocardial cells.

Text Links:
U C V 1 **M1-071**
U C V 2 MC-163

Figure M-M1-073
Urethral specimen showing intracellular cytoplasmic inclusions.

Text Link:
[U][C][V][1] M1-073

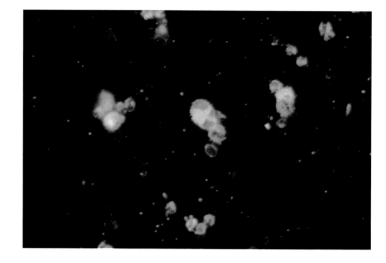

Figure M-M1-076
Intranuclear inclusion body.

Text Link:
[U][C][V][1] M1-076

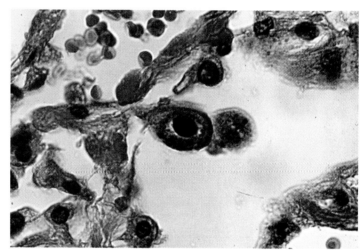

Figure M-M1-081
Ziehl-Nielsen stain of stool specimen showing acid fast oocysts.

Text Links:
[U][C][V][1] M1-081
[U][C][V][2] MC-166

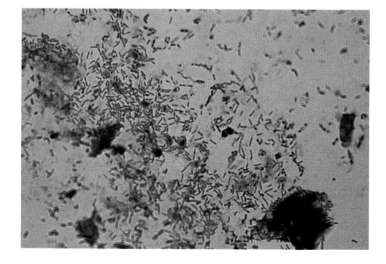

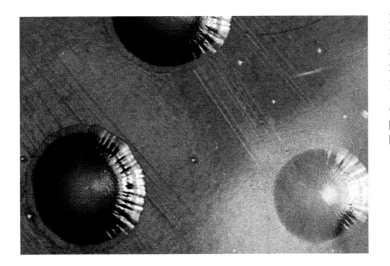

Figure M-M1-082
Black, tiny, dome-shaped colonies growing on a tellurite plate.

Text Links:
U C V 1 **M1-082**
U C V 2 MC-324

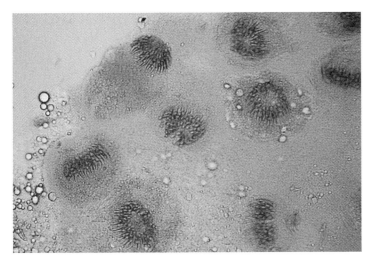

Figure M-M1-083
Multiple protoscoleces in cyst fluid.

Text Links:
U C V 1 **M1-083**
U C V 2 MC-167

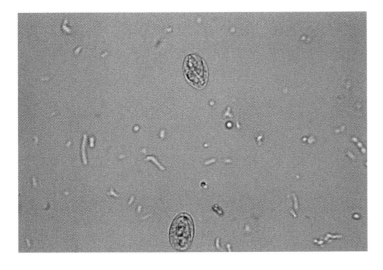

Figure M-M1-089A
Stool specimen showing protozoan cysts with four nuclei.

Text Links:
U C V 1 **M1-089**
U C V 2 MC-171

Figure M-M1-089B
Pear-shaped tropho-
zoite with two nuclei.

Text Links:
UCV1 **M1-089**
UCV2 MC-171

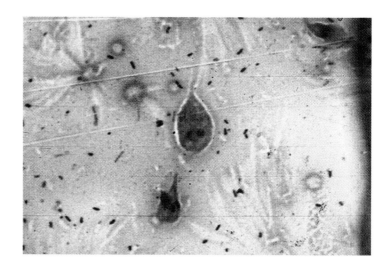

Figure M-M1-091
Gram-negative diplo-
cocci in a urethral
specimen.

Text Links:
UCV1 **M1-091**
UCV2 IM2-018

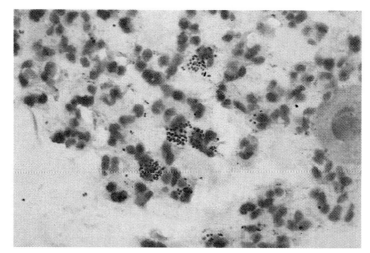

Figure M-M1-100
Multinucleated giant
cells undergoing bal-
looning degeneration.

Text Links:
UCV1 **M1-100**
UCV2 IM2-019

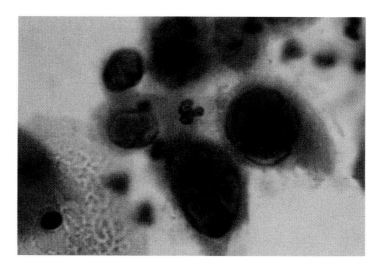

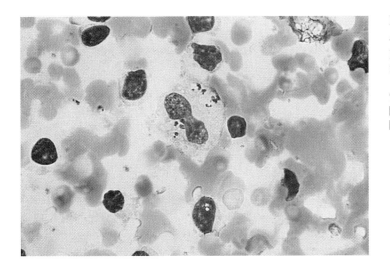

Figure M-M2-014A
Amastigote form of parasite within macrophages.

Text Links:
U C V 1 **M2-014**
U C V 2 MC-178

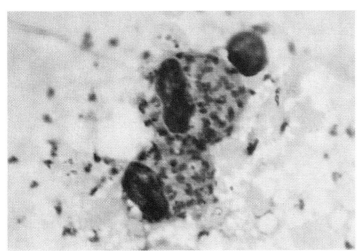

Figure M-M2-014B
Foamy macrophages filled with parasites.

Text Links:
U C V 1 **M2-014**
U C V 2 MC-178

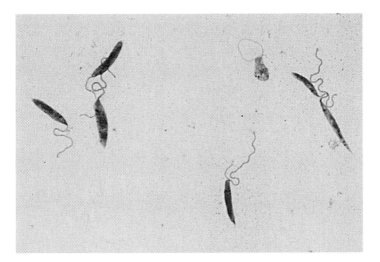

Figure M-M2-014C
Flagellated protozoan.

Text Links:
U C V 1 **M2-014**
U C V 2 MC-178

Figure M-M2-020
Adult worm obstruct-
ing a lymphatic
channel.

Text Link:
U C V 1 M2-020

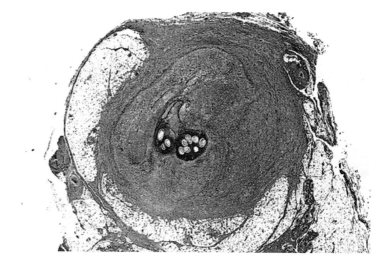

Figure M-M2-025
Non-septate hyphae
branching at right
angles.

Text Link:
U C V 1 M2-025

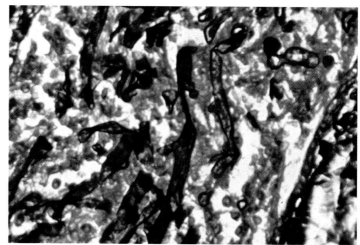

Figure M-M2-035A
Small α-hemolytic
colonies growing on
blood agar.

Text Links:
U C V 1 M2-035
U C V 2 IM2-025

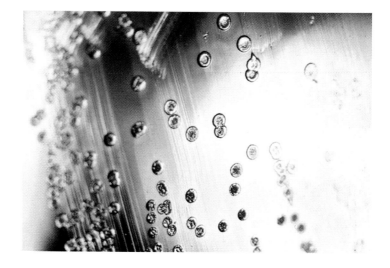

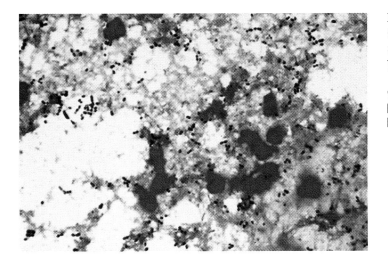

Figure M-M2-035B
Gram-positive diplo-
cocci seen in lung
biopsy.

Text Links:
⬜C⬜1 **M2-035**
⬜C⬜2 IM2-025

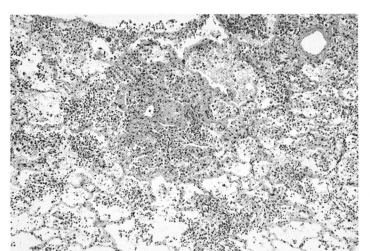

Figure M-M2-035C
Dense neutrophilic
infiltrate within
alveoli. Congested
septal capillaries.

Text Links:
⬜C⬜1 **M2-035**
⬜C⬜2 IM2-025

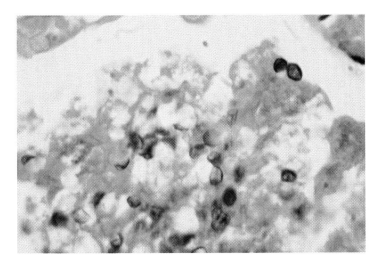

Figure M-M2-036A
Methenamine silver
stain of sputum
specimen demonstrat-
ing multiple cystic
organisms.

Text Link:
⬜C⬜1 **M2-036**

Figure M-M2-036B
Numerous parasitic cysts within alveolar exudates.

Text Link:
⬚U⬚C⬚V⬚1 M2-036

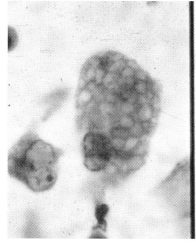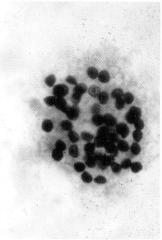

Figure M-M2-036C
Acellular, foamy eosinophilic exudate within alveoli.

Text Link:
⬚U⬚C⬚V⬚1 M2-036

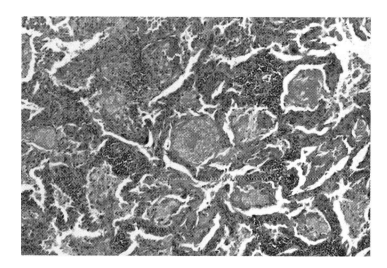

Figure M-M2-041
Intracytoplasmic inclusions within hippocampal neurons.

Text Links:
⬚U⬚C⬚V⬚1 M2-041
⬚U⬚C⬚V⬚2 MC-231

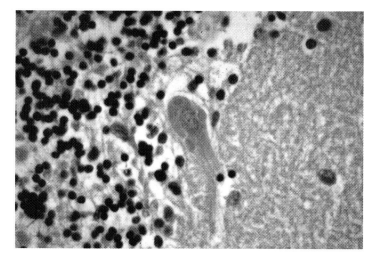

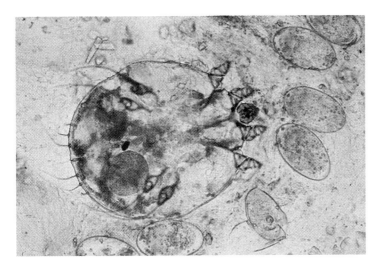

Figure M-M2-049
Skin burrow contents showing the female mite and surrounding eggs.

Text Links:
U C V 1 **M2-049**
U C V 2 MC-186

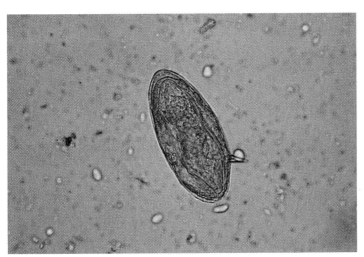

Figure M-M2-051
Trematode ovum with prominent lateral spine.

Text Link:
U C V 1 **M2-051**

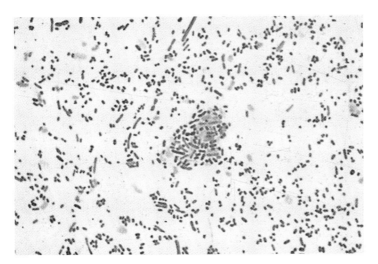

Figure M-M2-054A
Gram-negative rods.

Text Links:
U C V 1 **M2-054**
U C V 2 ER-026

Figure M-M2-054B
Round, pink colonies
growing on blood
agar.

Text Links:
⬜U⬜C⬜V⬜1 **M2-054**
⬜U⬜C⬜V⬜2 ER-026

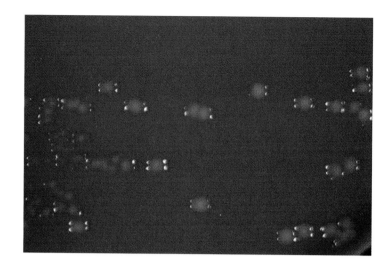

Figure M-M2-055
Chlamydospore aster-
oid body.

Text Link:
⬜U⬜C⬜V⬜1 **M2-055**

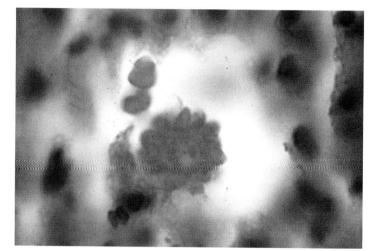

Figure M-M2-056
Rhabditiform larvae in
stool specimen.

Text Link:
⬜U⬜C⬜V⬜1 **M2-056**

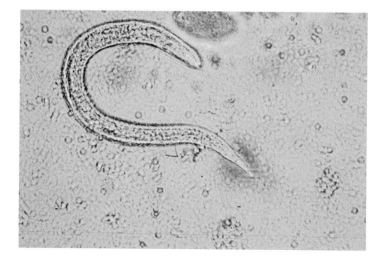

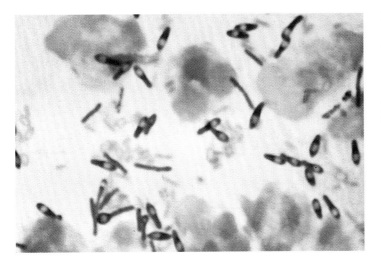

Figure M-M2-062
Gram-positive rods
with oval subterminal
and terminal spores.

Text Links:
UCV1 **M2-062**
UCV2 MC-232

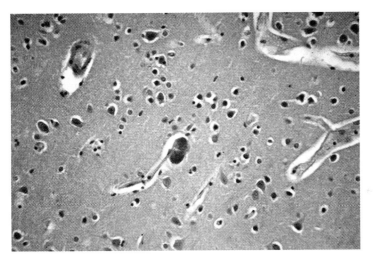

Figure M-M2-065
Crescent-shaped
trophozoites and cysts
in brain.

Text Links:
UCV1 **M2-065**
UCV2 MC-191

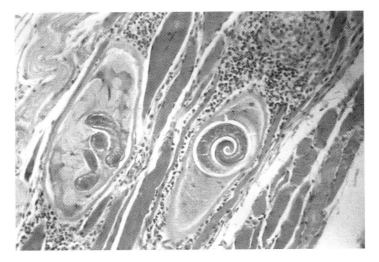

Figure M-M2-066
Encapsulated larvae
within skeletal
muscle.

Text Links:
UCV1 **M2-066**
UCV2 MC-192

Figure M-M2-068A
Ziehl-Nielsen stain
showing acid-fast
bacilli.

Text Links:
UCV1 **M2-068**
UCV2 IM2-029

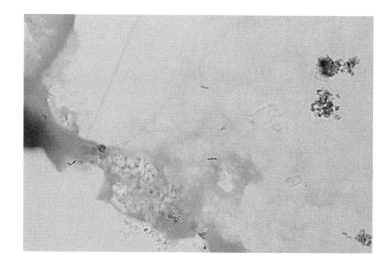

Figure M-M2-068B
Ziehl-Nielsen staining
of lymph node speci-
men showing clusters
of acid-fast bacilli.

Text Links:
UCV1 **M2-068**
UCV2 IM2-029

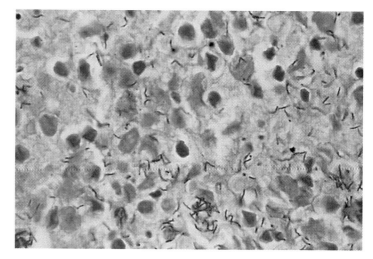

Figure M-M2-068C
Multinucleated giant
cell.

Text Links:
UCV1 **M2-068**
UCV2 IM2-029

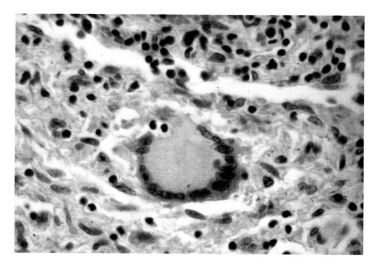

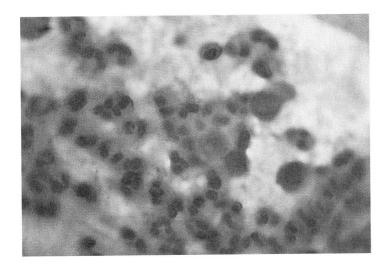

Figure M-M2-071
Gram stain of urethral discharge demonstrating numerous neutrophils.

Text Links:
U C V 1 **M2-071**
U C V 2 ER-027

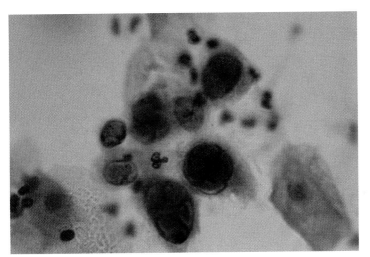

Figure M-M2-074
Multinucleated giant cells.

Text Links:
U C V 1 **M2-074**
U C V 2 PED-035

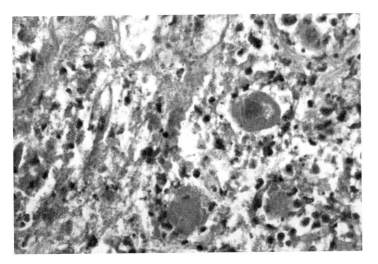

Figure M-M2-089
Dark intranuclear inclusion bodies.

Text Links:
U C V 1 **M2-089**
U C V 2 NEU-021

Figure M-M2-092
Gram stain of cerebrospinal fluid, showing many red stained cells.

Text Links:
UCV1 **M2-092**
UCV2 NEU-027

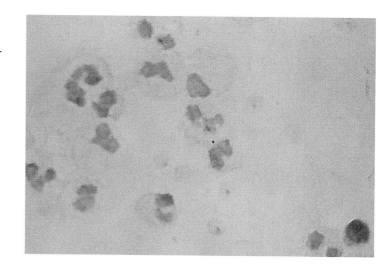

Figure M-M2-093
Bacterial colonies grown on chocolate agar, enriched with factors V and X.

Text Link:
UCV1 **M2-093**

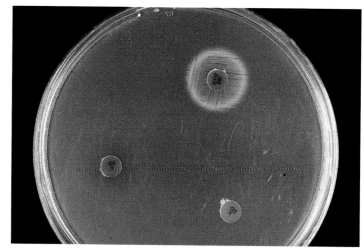

Figure M-M2-094
Cerebrospinal fluid stained with India ink, showing encapsulated organism.

Text Links:
UCV1 **M2-094**
UCV2 IM2-040

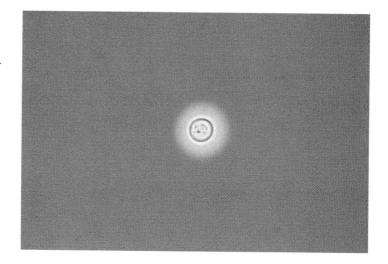

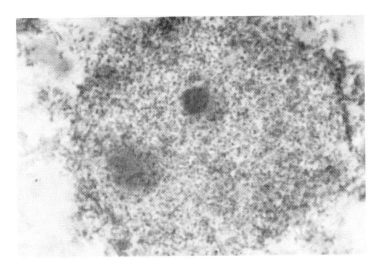

Figure M-M2-101
Epithelial cell covered
with bacteria.

Text Links:
UCV1 **M2-101**
UCV2 OB-001

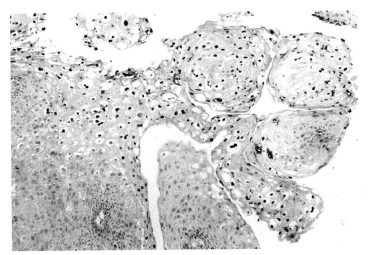

Figure M-M2-103
Cytoplasmic vacuoles
within squamous
epithelial cells.

Text Links:
UCV1 **M2-103**
UCV2 OB-011

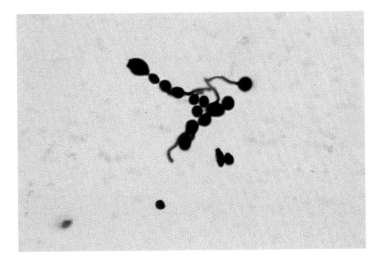

Figure M-P1-079
Germ-tube formation
in serum at 37°C.

Text Links:
UCV1 **P1-079**
UCV2 MC-100

Figure PG-A-002

Smooth-walled defect in midseptum due to defect in the foramen ovale.

Text Links:
UCV1 **A-002**
UCV2 SUR-001

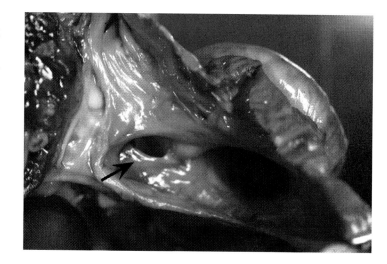

Figure PG-A-004

Narrowing of aortic lumen just distal to site of the ductus arteriosis. Aortic arch and vessels proximal to lesion are dilated.

Text Links:
UCV1 **A-004**
UCV2 SUR-002

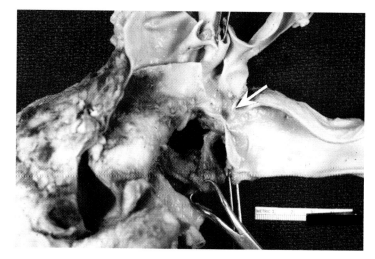

Figure PG-A-006

Abnormal communication between left pulmonary artery and aorta, just distal to origin of the left subclavian artery.

Text Links:
UCV1 **A-006**
UCV2 PED-001

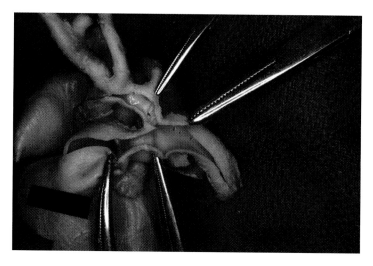

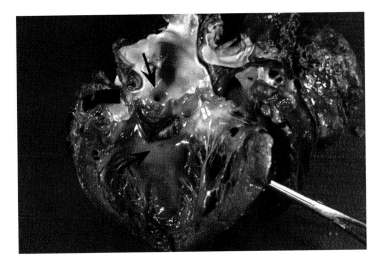

Figure PG-A-007
VSD viewed from the left ventricle with aorta overlying both the right and left ventricles. Not shown are sub pulmonary stenosis and hypertrophic right ventricle.

Text Links:
UCV1 **A-007**
UCV2 SUR-003

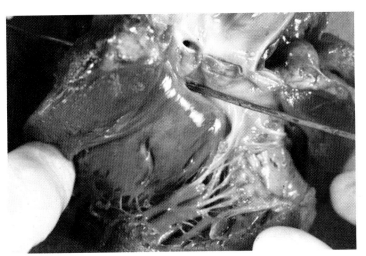

Figure PG-A-008
Perforation of perimembranous area of the ventricular septum just below the aortic valve.

Text Links:
UCV1 **A-008**
UCV2 PED-003

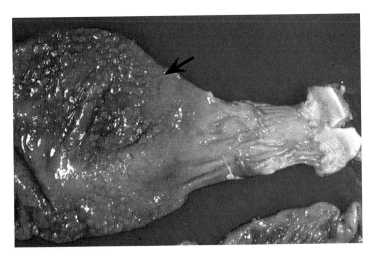

Figure PG-A-022
Striking dilation of proximal segment of colon with abrupt distal narrowing.

Text Links:
UCV1 **A-022**
UCV2 MC-312

Figure PG-A-024A
Gastric wall
perforation.

Text Links:
UCV1 **A-024**
UCV2 SUR-014

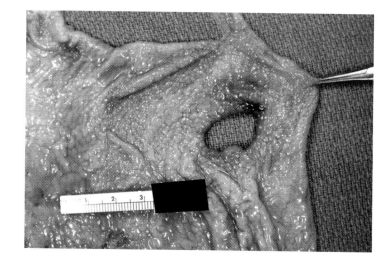

Figure PG-A-024B
Defect and hemor-
rhage extending
through the stomach
wall along the greater
curvature.

Text Links:
UCV1 **A-024**
UCV2 SUR-014

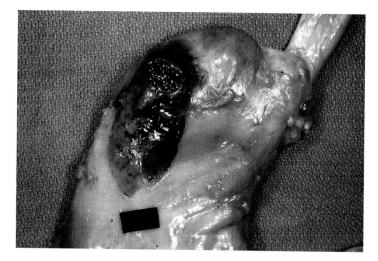

Figure PG-A-025
Dilated, tortuous
veins in the
submucosa at the
cardio-esophageal
junction.

Text Links:
UCV1 **A-025**
UCV2 SUR-016

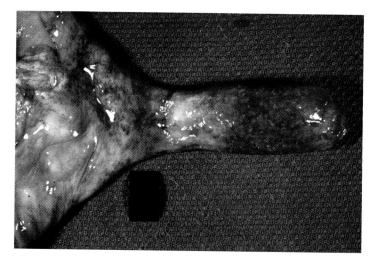

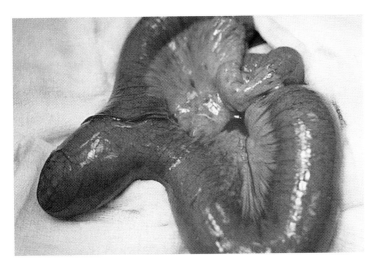

Figure PG-A-032
Tubular outpouching of the small intestine.

Text Links:
UCV1 **A-032**
UCV2 PED-010

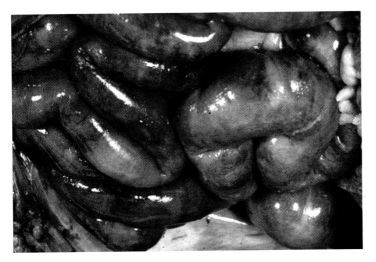

Figure PG-A-033
Purple, subserosal ecchymotic discoloration and edematous thickened intestinal wall.

Text Links:
UCV1 **A-033**
UCV2 SUR-032

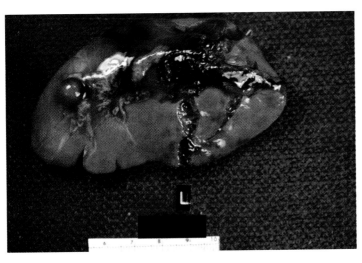

Figure PG-A-038
Capsular tear with subcapsular hemorrhage on superior aspect of the spleen.

Text Links:
UCV1 **A-038**
UCV2 SUR-034

Figure PG-A-047
Multiple smooth, round calculi within the renal pelvis and calyces.

Text Links:
UCV1 **A-047**
UCV2 ER-030

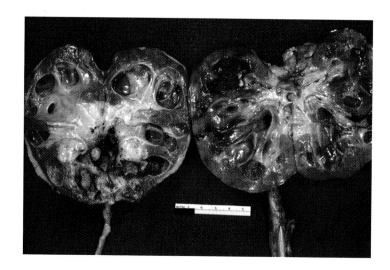

Figure PG-A-049
Well-circumscribed mass attached to CNVIII, lying within cerebellar-pontine angle.

Text Links:
UCV1 **A-049**
UCV2 MC-368

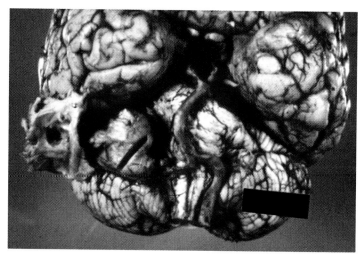

Figure PG-A-052
Irregularly-shaped, hemorrhagic mass infiltrating the right temporal lobe.

Text Links:
UCV1 **A-052**
UCV2 NEU-002

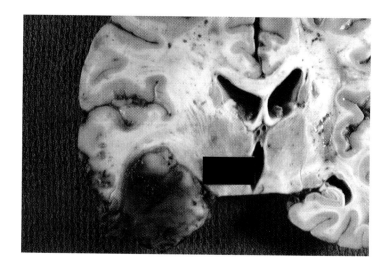

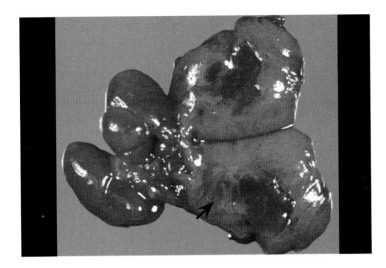

Figure PG-BC-013
Well-circumscribed, soft tan nodule with central cystification within a delicate capsule.

Text Links:
UCV1 **BC-013**
UCV2 IM1-022

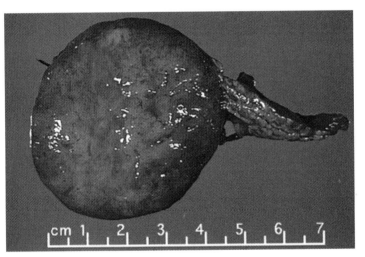

Figure PG-BC-026A
Circumscribed, fleshy, gray pink mass with adjacent compressed adrenal gland.

Text Links:
UCV1 **BC-026**
UCV2 SUR-007

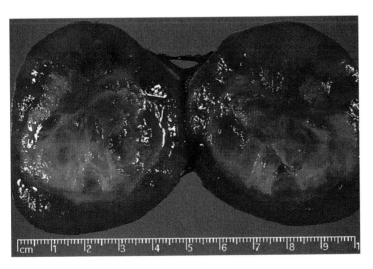

Figure PG-BC-026B
Large tumor with areas of hemorrhage, cyst formation and focal necrosis.

Text Links:
UCV1 **BC-026**
UCV2 SUR-007

Figure PG-BC-083
Heavy, firm, red and boggy lungs.

Text Links:
UCV1 **BC-083**
UCV2 PED-041

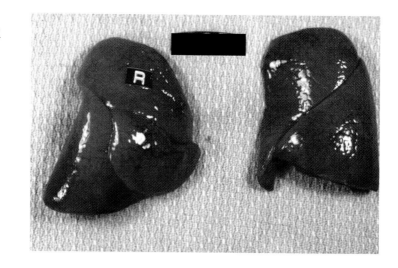

Figure PG-BC-085
Pseudohypertrophy due to fibrofatty replacement of skeletal muscle.

Text Links:
UCV1 **BC-085**
UCV2 PED-049

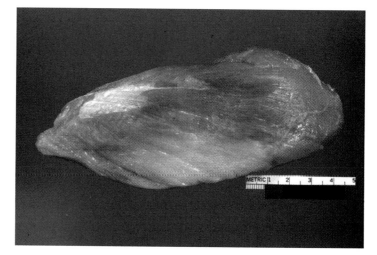

Figure PG-BC-086
Brown discoloration of the mamillary bodies due to hemosiderin deposition.

Text Links:
UCV1 **BC-086**
UCV2 PSY-003

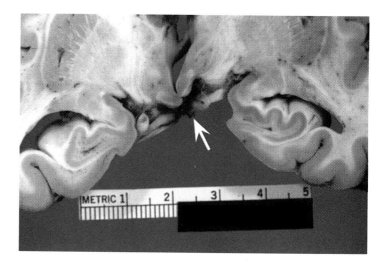

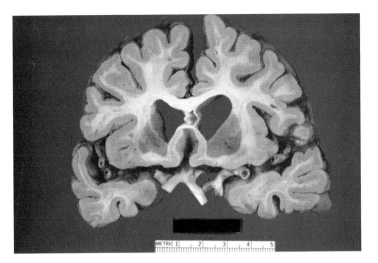

Figure PG-BS-005
Diffuse cortical atrophy with mild enlargement of the lateral ventricles, widened sulci and narrowed gyri.

Text Links:
U C V 1 **BS-005**
U C V 2 PSY-002

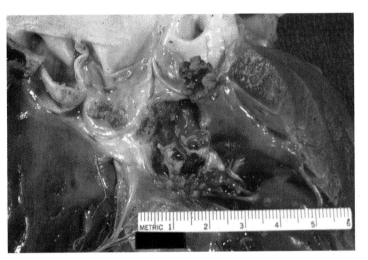

Figure PG-M1-001
Multiple friable vegetations infiltrating the cusps and chordae tendinae of tricuspid valve.

Text Links:
U C V 1 **M1-001**
U C V 2 IM2-001

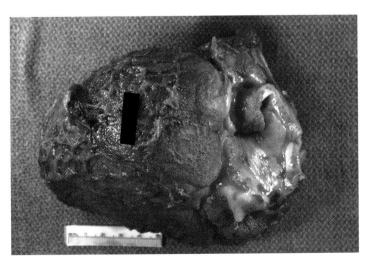

Figure PG-M1-003
Shaggy, fibrinous exudate overlying the epicardial surface facing the pericardium.

Text Links:
U C V 1 **M1-003**
U C V 2 IM1-012

Figure PG-M1-005A
Small, firm vegetations along the atrioventricular valve cusps. Fragile, elongated chordae tendinae.

Text Links:
UCV1 **M1-005**
UCV2 IM2-002

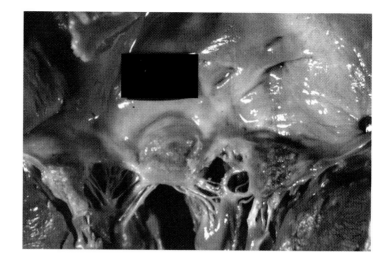

Figure PG-M1-033
Dusky gray discoloration and focal hemorrhages of the colonic mucosa.

Text Links:
UCV1 **M1-033**
UCV2 PED-043

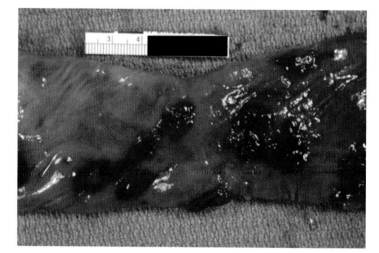

Figure PG-M1-035
Well-demarcated mucosal defect with smooth borders and hemorrhagic base, extending into submucosa.

Text Links:
UCV1 **M1-035**
UCV2 IM1-038

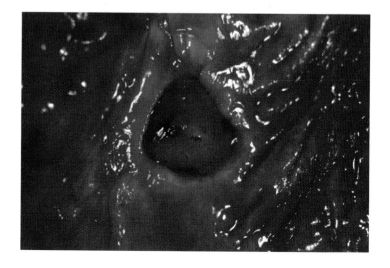

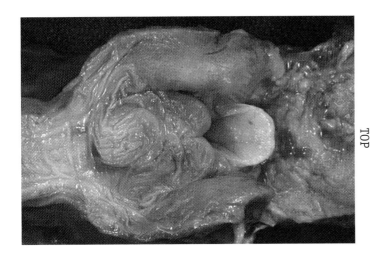

Figure PG-M1-087
Red, markedly edematous epiglottis and surrounding soft tissues with resultant airway obstruction.

Text Links:
U C V 1 **M1-087**
U C V 2 ER-025

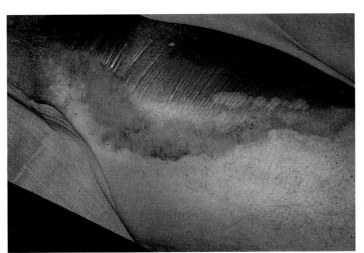

Figure PG-M1-088
Well-demarcated area of fluid- and gas-filled blisters at edge of necrotic skin with surrounding erythema and edema.

Text Link:
U C V 1 **M1-088**

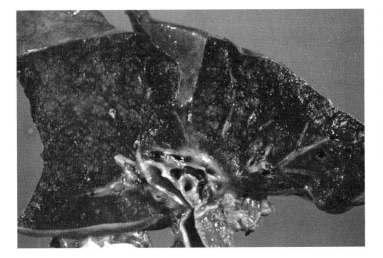

Figure PG-M2-035
Red, boggy, congested lung parenchyma with peri-bronchial tan yellow nodular consolidation.

Text Links:
U C V 1 **M2-035**
U C V 2 IM2-025

Figure PG-M2-067
Small, yellow, well-demarcated centrally caseating nodules disseminated throughout the spleen.

Text Link:
UCV1 M2-067

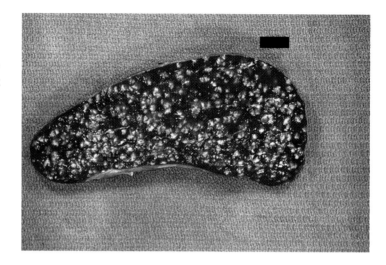

Figure PG-M2-068A
Diffusely replaced lung parenchyma with tan white nodules cavitations and areas of honey comb fibrosis.

Text Links:
UCV1 M2-068
UCV2 IM2-029

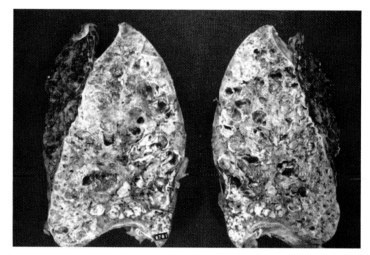

Figure PG-M2-068B
Large subpleural apical cavitations and scattered white chalky nodules.

Text Links:
UCV1 M2-068B
UCV2 IM2-029B

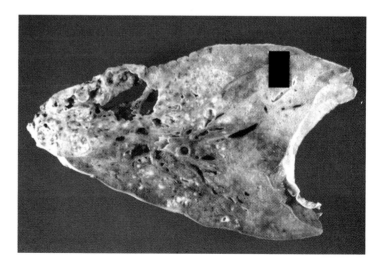

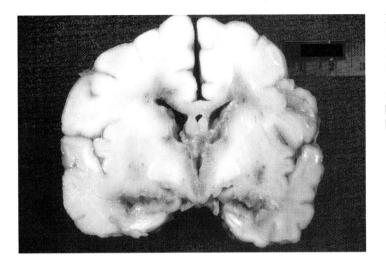

Figure PG-M2-079
Swollen brain parenchyma with opaque meninges.

Text Links:
UCV1 **M2-079**
UCV2 MC-250

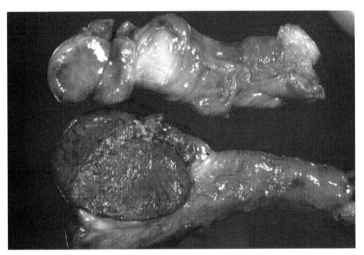

Figure PG-M2-082
Shrunken red, edematous testicle (compare with normal on the bottom).

Text Links:
UCV1 **M2-082**
UCV2 MC-366

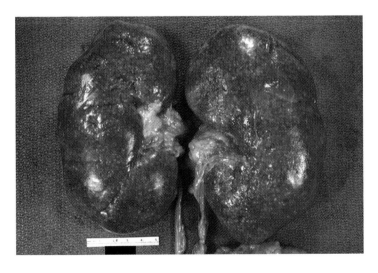

Figure PG-M2-086A
Diffuse microabscesses of the renal cortex.

Text Links:
UCV1 **M2-086**
UCV2 ER-031

Figure PG-M2-086B
Microabscesses and hemorrhage of the renal parenchyma extending through medullary pyramids to cortex.

Text Links:
UCV1 **M2-086**
UCV2 ER-031

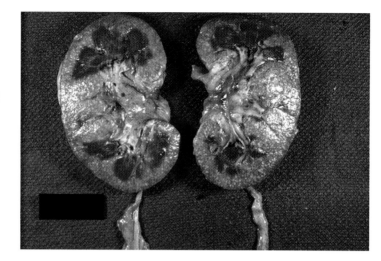

Figure PG-M2-092A
Opaque meninges with creamy, purulent exudates overlying the cerebral convexities.

Text Links:
UCV1 **M2-092**
UCV2 NEU-027

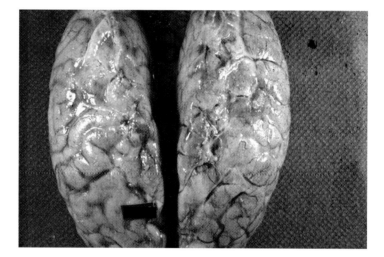

Figure PG-M2-092B
Purulent exudates overlying the temporal lobes, brainstem and cerebellum.

Text Links:
UCV1 **M2-092**
UCV2 NEU-027

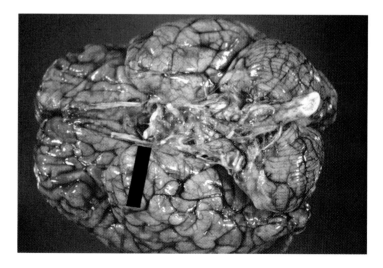

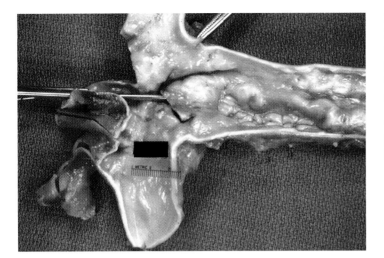

Figure PG-P1-001
Longitudinal tear in the descending thoracic aorta just distal to origin of the left subclavian artery.

Text Links:
Ⓤ Ⓒ Ⓥ 1 **P1-001**
Ⓤ Ⓒ Ⓥ 2 ER-001

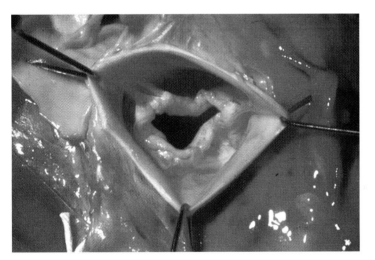

Figure PG-P1-003
Deformation and calcium deposition of the aortic valve cusps.

Text Links:
Ⓤ Ⓒ Ⓥ 1 **P1-003**
Ⓤ Ⓒ Ⓥ 2 IM1-002

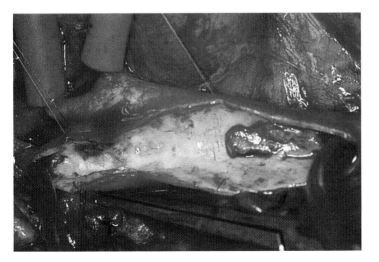

Figure PG-P1-004A
Large, loosely adherent yellow plaque seen in the common carotid artery.

Text Link:
Ⓤ Ⓒ Ⓥ 1 **P1-004**

Figure PG-P1-004B
Yellow-gray fibrofatty plaque adherent to the intima of aortic lumen.

Text Link:
U C V 1 **P1-004**

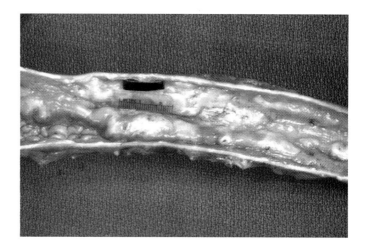

Figure PG-P1-006
Large gray pedunculated mass arising from the fossa ovalis and occluding the left atrium.

Text Links:
U C V 1 **P1-006**
U C V 2 IM1-003

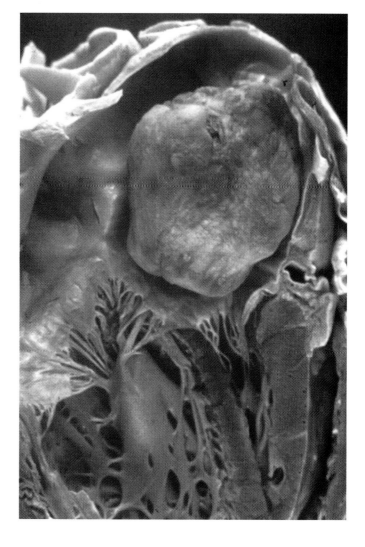

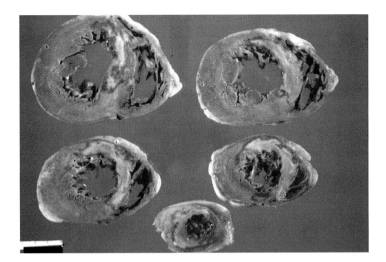

Figure PG-P1-007
Pale yellow-gray lesion with hyperemic border in the inter-ventricular septum of heart.

Text Links:
U C V 1 **P1-007**
U C V 2 ER-002

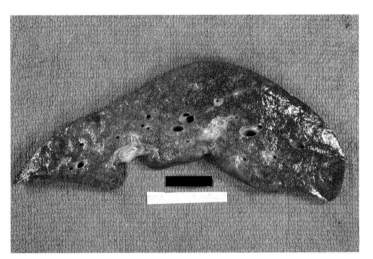

Figure PG-P1-010A
Nutmeg pattern of hepatic congestion due to centrilobular necrosis.

Text Links:
U C V 1 **P1-010**
U C V 2 IM1-004

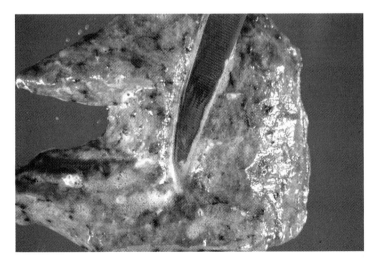

Figure PG-P1-010B
Red congested lungs with pink frothy fluid expressable from parenchyma.

Text Links:
U C V 1 **P1-010**
U C V 2 IM1-004

Figure PG-P1-013
Enlarged, flabby heart with marked bi-ventricular dilation.

Text Links:
UCV1 **P1-013**
UCV2 IM1-006

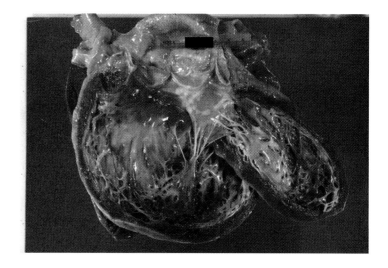

Figure PG-P1-016
Hypertrophic septum impinging on the left ventricular outflow tract.

Text Links:
UCV1 **P1-016**
UCV2 IM1-007

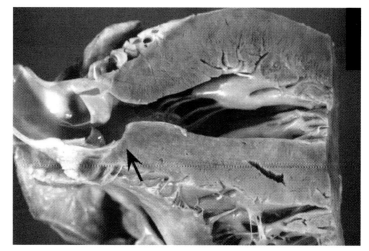

Figure PG-P1-018
Multiple small petechial hemorrhages on the cortical surface of kidney.

Text Links:
UCV1 **P1-018**
UCV2 ER-005

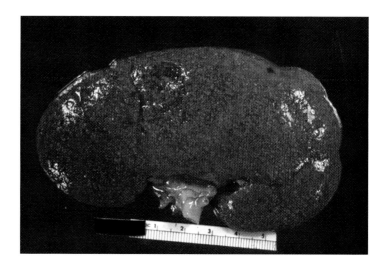

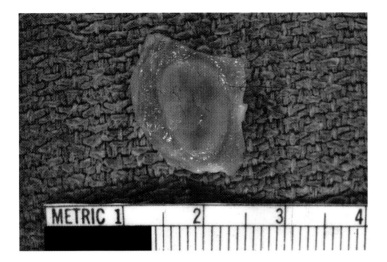

Figure PG-P1-054
Solitary, spherical, circumscribed fleshy pink-red mass within normal thyroid tissue.

Text Links:
U C V 1 **P1-058**
U C V 2 MC-338

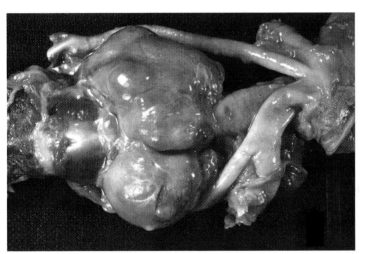

Figure PG-P1-060
Irregular, dark blue nodules diffusely replacing the thyroid visible on the anterior surface.

Text Links:
U C V 1 **P1-060**
U C V 2 MC-094

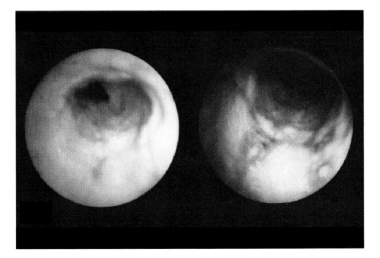

Figure PG-P1-077
Replacement of normal smooth esophageal white pink mucosa with patchy red granular mucosa (normal on left).

Text Links:
U C V 1 **P1-077**
U C V 2 MC-098

Figure PG-P1-079
Yellow-white pseudomembrane overlying an erythematous esophageal mucosa.

Text Links:
U C V 1 **P1-079**
U C V 2 MC-100

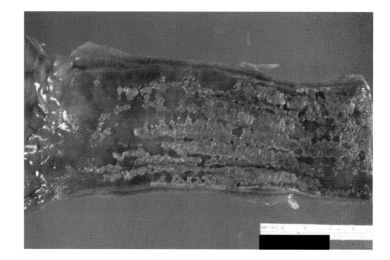

Figure PG-P1-082
Markedly dilated pancreatic ducts, obstructed by calculous deposits.

Text Links:
U C V 1 **P1-082**
U C V 2 IM1-029

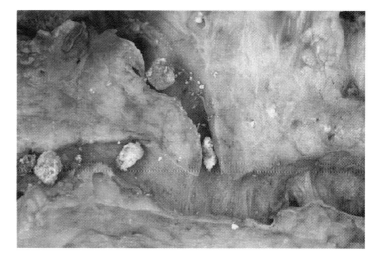

Figure PG-P1-086
Mucosal openings to multiple diverticuli within adjacent discolored and edematous (inflamed) mucosa.

Text Links:
U C V 1 **P1-086**
U C V 2 IM1-031

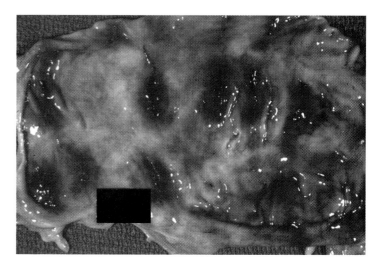

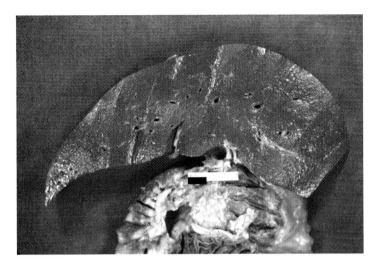

Figure PG-P1-090
Rusty discoloration of the liver.

Text Links:
U C V 1 **P1-090**
U C V 2 IM1-033

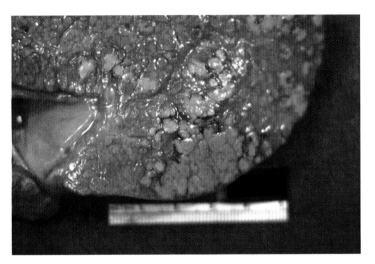

Figure PG-P1-091A
Diffuse nodularity and fibrosis on the cut-surface of the liver.

Text Links:
U C V 1 **P1-091**
U C V 2 IM1-034

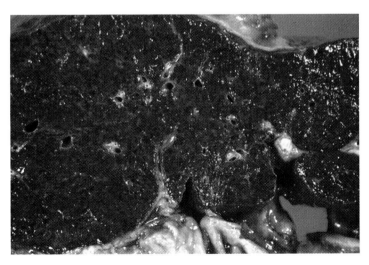

Figure PG-P1-091B
Dark green cholestatic liver with a faintly nodular surface.

Text Links:
U C V 1 **P1-091**
U C V 2 IM1-034

Figure PG-P1-096
Multiple discrete, white, irregularly shaped masses in the liver.

Text Link:
⬛UCV1⬛ **P1-096**

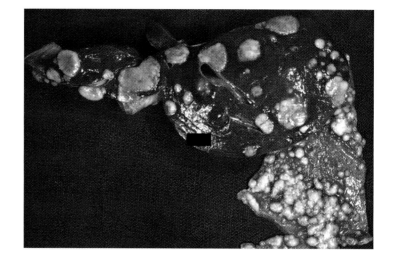

Figure PG-P1-102
Red, granular mucosa and pseudopolyps.

Text Links:
⬛UCV1⬛ **P1-102**
⬛UCV2⬛ IM1-040

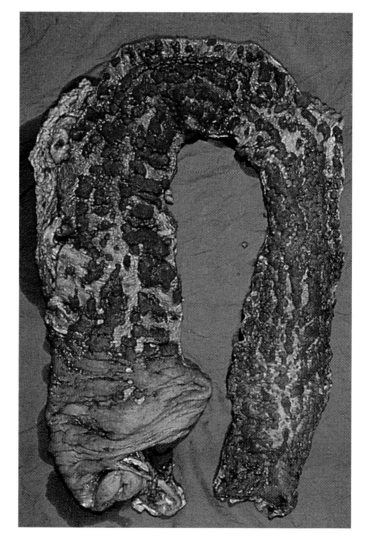

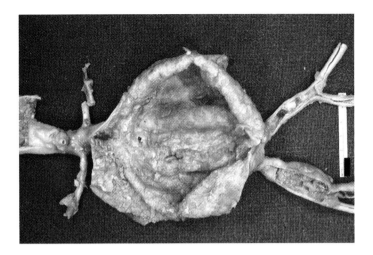

Figure PG-P2-001
Large saccular swelling of the abdominal aorta just proximal to iliac bifurcation.

Text Links:
UCV1 **P2-001**
UCV2 ER-015

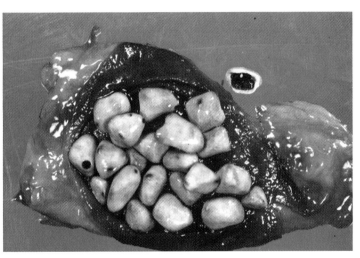

Figure PG-P2-002
Cholelithiasis, with multifaceted pale yellow calculi within the lumen of the gall-bladder, can lead to acute cholecystitis in cases of outflow obstruction.

Text Links:
UCV1 **P2-002**
UCV2 SUR-017

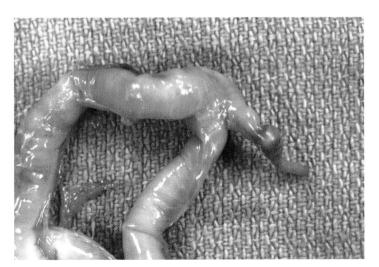

Figure PG-P2-003
Appendix with dusky hemorrhagic green discolored serosa attached to the cecum.

Text Links:
UCV1 **P2-003**
UCV2 SUR-020

Figure PG-P2-004
Fungating mass replacing the cecal wall and constricting the lumen.

Text Link:
[U][C][V][1] **P2-004**

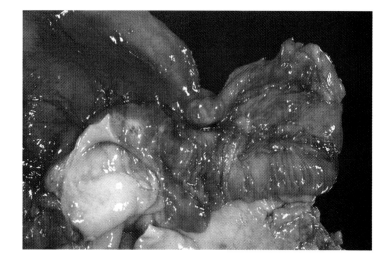

Figure PG-P2-005A
Gray-white irregular mass obliterating the esophageal lumen and eroding into the trachea.

Text Links:
[U][C][V][1] **P2-005**
[U][C][V][2] SUR-022

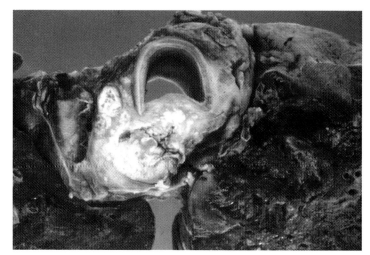

Figure PG-P2-005B
Gray-white mass with focal hemorrhage, narrowing the lumen of the esophagus.

Text Links:
[U][C][V][1] **P2-005**
[U][C][V][2] SUR-022

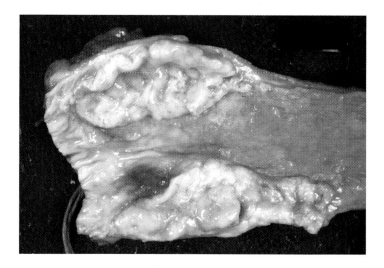

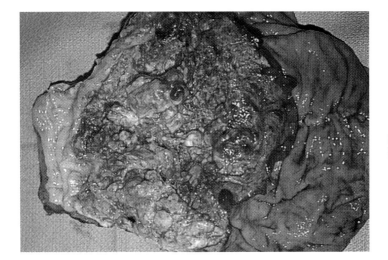

Figure PG-P2-006
Large hemorrhagic mass with destruction of mucosal folds in the antrum of the stomach.

Text Links:
⬜C⬜V⬜1 **P2-006**
⬜C⬜V⬜2 SUR-025

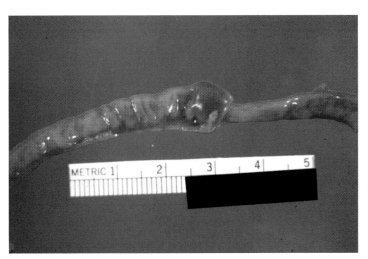

Figure PG-P2-009
Telescoping of a proximal segment of small bowel from the ileocecal region into an immediately distal segment, with subsequent submucosal hemorrhage.

Text Links:
⬜C⬜V⬜1 **P2-009**
⬜C⬜V⬜2 ER-017

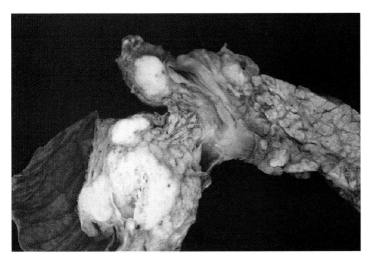

Figure PG-P2-010
Firm nodular mass with irregular borders involving the head of the pancreas.

Text Links:
⬜C⬜V⬜1 **P2-010**
⬜C⬜V⬜2 SUR-033

Figure PG-P2-045
"Tree bark" appearance; longitudinal streaks of inflammation separated by white areas of intimal fibrosis (atherosclerosis is present as well).

Text Links:
UCV1 **P2-045**
UCV2 MC-190

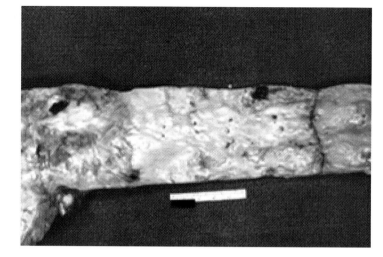

Figure PG-P2-048
Pale, edematous renal cortices with congested medullary regions making cortico-medullary junction pronounced.

Text Links:
UCV1 **P2-048**
UCV2 IM2-032

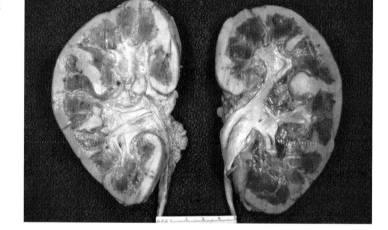

Figure PG-P2-052
Peri-urethral prostatic hyperplasia with prominent hyperplastic nodule in median lobe, protruding into the bladder.

Text Links:
UCV1 **P2-052**
UCV2 SUR-035

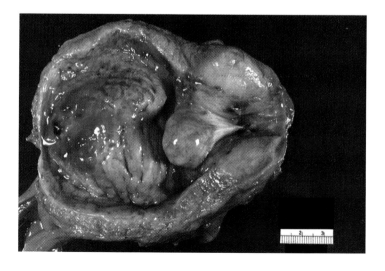

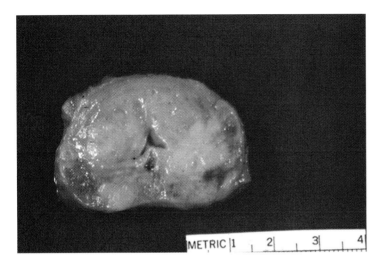

Figure PG-P2-063
Ill-defined firm tan yellow nodules with predilection for periphery of the prostate (note absence of BPH).

Text Links:
U C V 1 **P2-063**
U C V 2 SUR-037

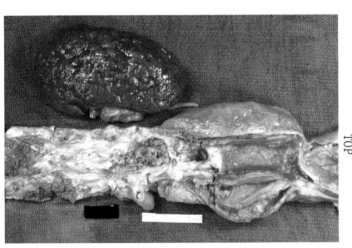

Figure PG-P2-066
Shrunken kidney with a granular capsule adjacent to aorta with atherosclerosis.

Text Links:
U C V 1 **P2-066**
U C V 2 IM2-038

TOP

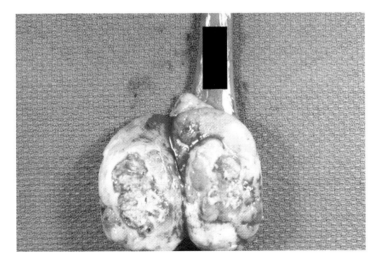

Figure PG-P2-067
Nodular gray-white mass replacing the testes.

Text Links:
U C V 1 **P2-067**
U C V 2 SUR-039

Figure PG-P2-081
Voluminous lungs
with pan-lobular
dilated airspaces most
pronounced in the
upper lobes.

Text Links:
U C V 1 **P2-081**
U C V 2 IM2-046

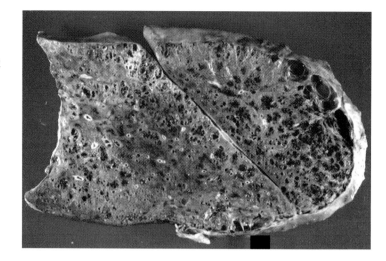

Figure PG-P2-085
Large gray-white mass
at the base of the
lower left lobe,
obstructing the left
bronchi.

Text Links:
U C V 1 **P2-085**
U C V 2 SUR-050

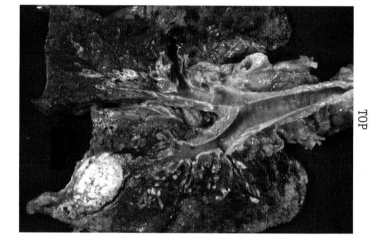

TOP

Figure PG-P2-086
White-gray plaque
like mass encasing
the lung most pro-
nounced at the lung
base.

Text Link:
U C V 1 **P2-086**

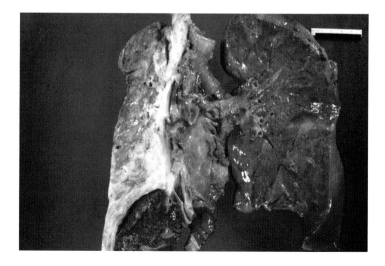

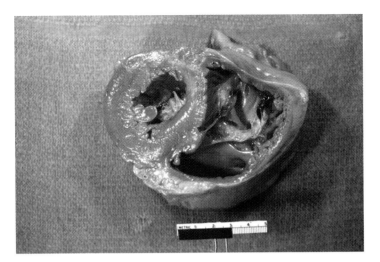

Figure PG-P2-090
Hypertrophic and dilated right ventricle.

Text Links:
UCV1 **P2-090**
UCV2 MC-214

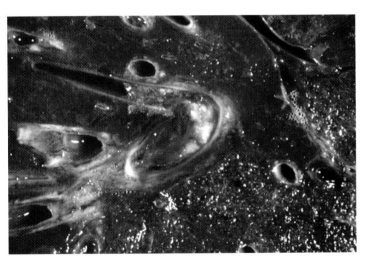

Figure PG-P2-091
Large, white, hemorrhagic clot obstructing the lumen of pulmonary artery.

Text Links:
UCV1 **P2-091**
UCV2 ER-046

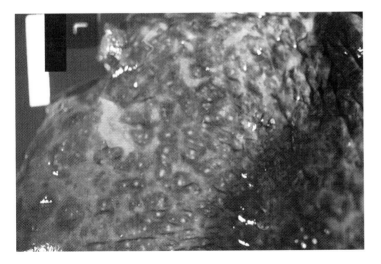

Figure PG-P2-093
Dense, small, blackened nodules just under the pleural surface of the lung.

Text Links:
UCV1 **P2-093**
UCV2 IM2-049

Figure PG-P3-006
Irregular, gray, cystic, calcified mass superior to the pituitary gland.

Text Links:
[UCV1] **P3-006**
[UCV2] NEU-007

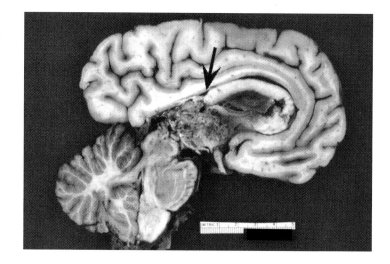

Figure PG-P3-010
Collection of blood overlying the dura mater and compressing the underlying brain parenchyma.

Text Links:
[UCV1] **P3-010**
[UCV2] SUR-040

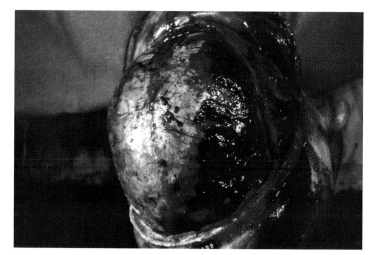

Figure PG-P3-012
Irregularly colored mass with hemorrhage, cysts and necrosis, infiltrating both cerebral hemispheres.

Text Links:
[UCV1] **P3-012**
[UCV2] NEU-019

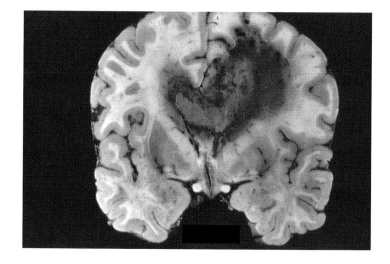

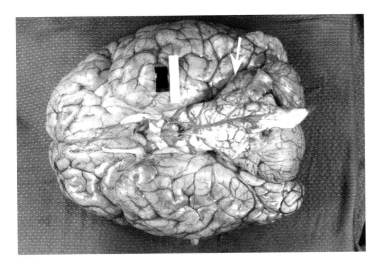

Figure PG-P3-018
Large protruding mass in the cerebellum involving the pons.

Text Links:
UCV1 **P3-018**
UCV2 NEU-024

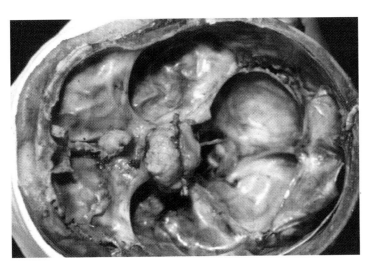

Figure PG-P3-020
Round, smooth gray masses attached to the meninges.

Text Links:
UCV1 **P3-020**
UCV2 MC-249

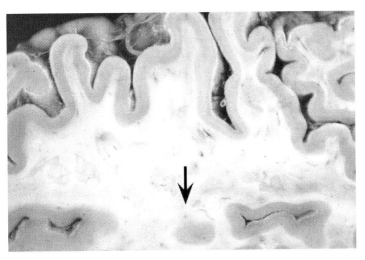

Figure PG-P3-023
Multiple discrete, well-demarcated gray plaques throughout the white matter.

Text Links:
UCV1 **P3-023**
UCV2 NEU-029

Figure PG-P3-026
Large, lobulated hem-
orrhagic mass obliter-
ating the left adrenal
gland, invading into
the renal parenchyma
and impinging on the
descending aorta.

Text Links:
UCV1 **P3-026**
UCV2 NEU-032

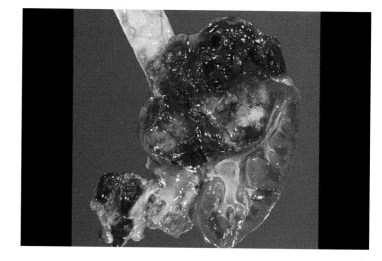

Figure PG-P3-031
Diffuse blood staining
the inferior surfaces
of the brainstem,
cerebellum, and
cerebral hemispheres.

Text Links:
UCV1 **P3-031**
UCV2 MC-264

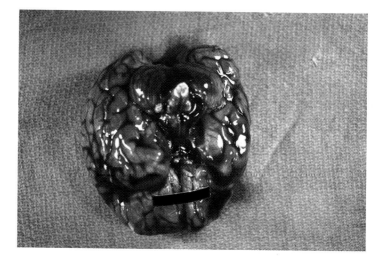

Figure PG-P3-032
Large well-demarcated
accumulation of
clotted blood
beneath the dura,
confined by dural
attachments.

Text Links:
UCV1 **P3-032**
UCV2 ER-035

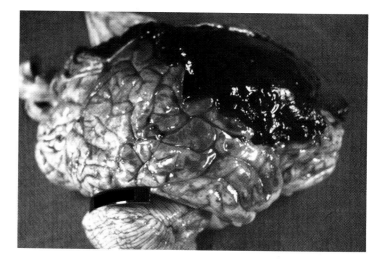

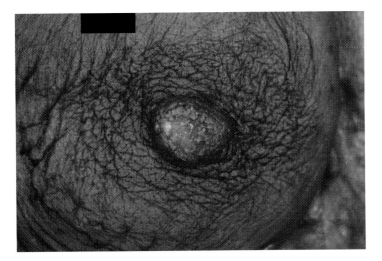

Figure PG-P3-042
Erosion and crusting of the nipple.

Text Links:
U C V 1 **P3-042**
U C V 2 MC-275

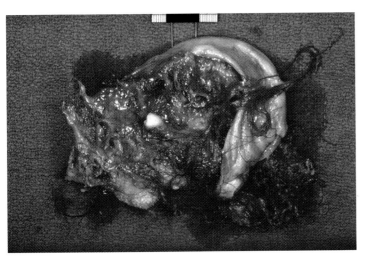

Figure PG-P3-055
Cystic ovarian mass containing matted hair, sebaceous material and a tooth.

Text Links:
U C V 1 **P3-055**
U C V 2 OB-017

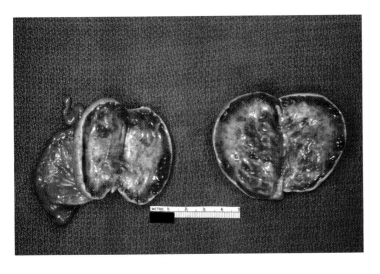

Figure PG-P3-056
Bilateral enlarged ovaries with multiple subcortical cysts.

Text Links:
U C V 1 **P3-056**
U C V 2 OB-020

Figure PG-P3-058
Multiple firm circumscribed, homogenous, yellowish nodules in the myometrium and protruding into endometrial cavity.

Text Links:
UCV1 **P3-058**
UCV2 OB-028

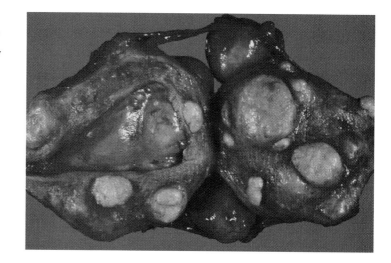

Figure PG-P3-059
Large fleshy tan mass in the myometrium with areas of hemorrhage softening and focal necrosis.

Text Link:
UCV1 **P3-059**

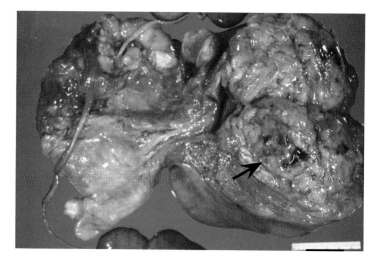

Figure PG-P3-073
Erosion of the articular cartilage and small osteophytes and subchondral sclerosis within the knee joint.

Text Links:
UCV1 **P3-073**
UCV2 SUR-044

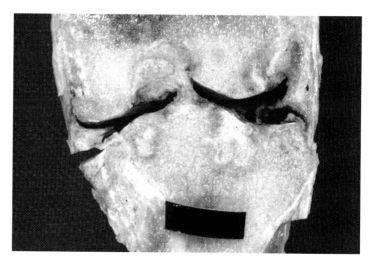

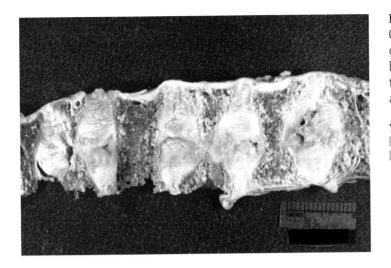

Figure PG-P3-085
Compression fractures of the veterbral bodies secondary to thinning of cortex and trabeculae.

Text Links:
U C V 1 **P3-085**
U C V 2 MC-223

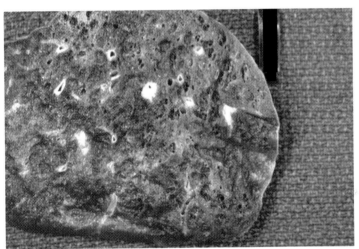

Figure PG-P3-089
Pulmonary fibrosis with a honeycomb appearance beneath the pleura (non-specific)

Text Links:
U C V 1 **P3-089**
U C V 2 MC-226

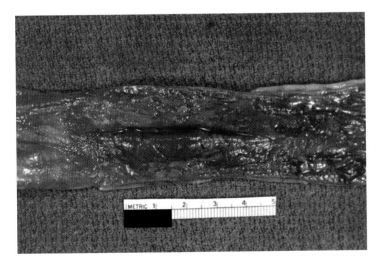

Figure PG-PH-031
Gray-green fibrinous layer adherent to the colonic mucosa.

Text Links:
U C V 1 **PH-031**
U C V 2 MC-110

Figure PM-A-069
Intracytoplasmic inclusion consisting of electron dense homogenous core surrounded by halo. Grossly substantia nigra appears pale due to depigmented neurons.

Text Links:
UCV1 A-069
UCV2 NEU-034

Figure PM-BC-003
Cells in a pituitary adenoma with positive cytoplasmic staining for growth hormone.

Text Links:
UCV1 BC-003
UCV2 MC-084

Figure PM-BC-009A
Pancreatic alpha cells with multiple electron dense, spherical cytoplasmic granules.

Text Links:
UCV1 BC-009
UCV2 IM1-020

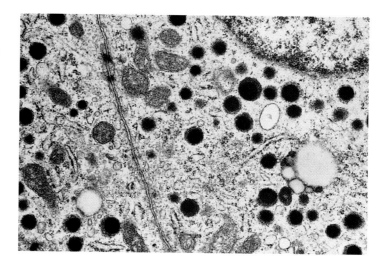

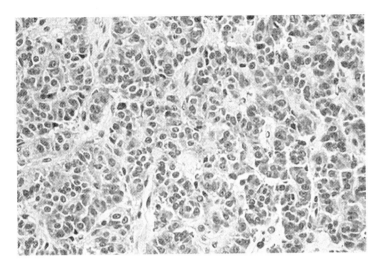

Figure PM-BC-009B
Proliferation of small, uniform, plasmacytoid pancreatic alpha cells.

Text Links:
UCV1 **BC-009**
UCV2 IM1-020

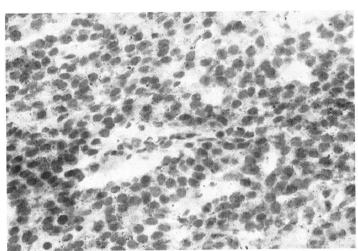

Figure PM-BC-013
Diffuse hyperplasia of the parathyroid chief cells with decreased extra and intracellular fat.

Text Links:
UCV1 **BC-013**
UCV2 IM1-022

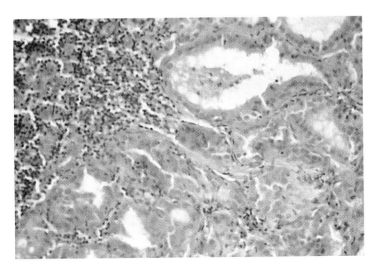

Figure PM-BC-014
Small follicles lined with hyperplastic epithelium. There is scant colloid and a lymphocytic infiltrate.

Text Links:
UCV1 **BC-014**
UCV2 MC-090

Figure PM-BC-026
Nests of large polygonal cells with abundant purplish cytoplasm, surrounded by a vascular stroma.

Text Links:
UCV1 **BC-026**
UCV2 SUR-007

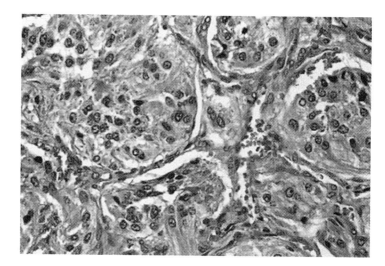

Figure PM-BC-085
Fatty infiltration of skeletal muscle.

Text Links:
UCV1 **BC-085**
UCV2 PED-049

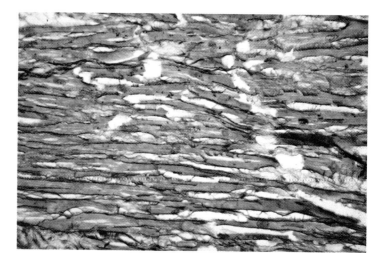

Figure PM-BC-094
Negatively birefringent long needle-shaped crystals.

Text Links:
UCV1 **BC-094**
UCV2 IM2-052

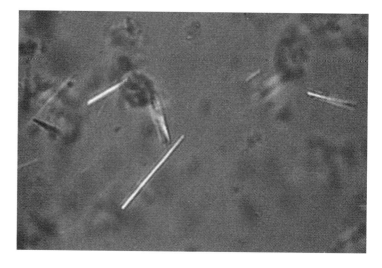

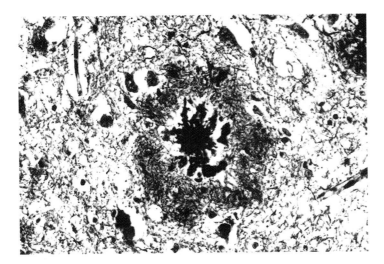

Figure PM-BS-005A
Coarse, filamentous aggregates of abnormal protein in the cytoplasm of neurons (neurofibrillary tangles).

Text Links:
U C V 1 **BS-005**
U C V 2 PSY-002

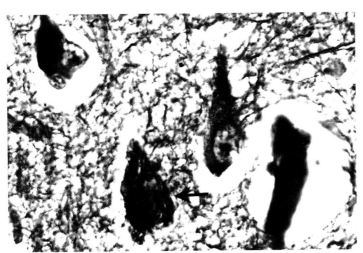

Figure PM-BS-005B
Extracellular aggregates of dystrophic neuritis surrounding amyloid core in brain tissue (neuritic plaques).

Text Links:
U C V 1 **BS-005**
U C V 2 PSY-002

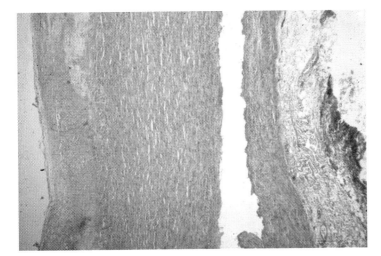

Figure PM-P1-001
Longitudinal tear in the tunica media of the aorta.

Text Links:
U C V 1 **P1-001**
U C V 2 ER-001

Figure PM-P1-004A
Intimal plaque con-
sisting of a fibrous
cap, necrotic core,
cholesterol clefts and
calcification.

Text Link:
UCVT1 P1-004

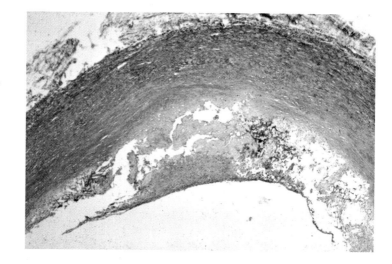

Figure PM-P1-004B
Intimal plaque con-
sisting of a fibrous
cap, necrotic core and
foam cells.

Text Link:
UCVT1 P1-004

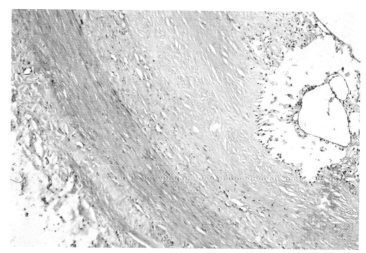

Figure PM-P1-007
Brightly eosinophilic
wavy cardiac muscle
fibers. Occasional
deeply-stained trans-
verse bands of my-
ocytes (contraction
band necrosis).

Text Links:
UCVT1 P1-007
UCVT2 ER-002

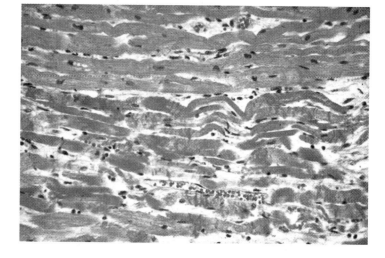

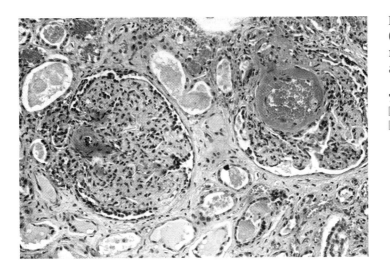

Figure PM-P1-018
Glomeruli with fibrinoid necrosis of arterioles.

Text Links:
U C V 1 **P1-018**
U C V 2 ER-005

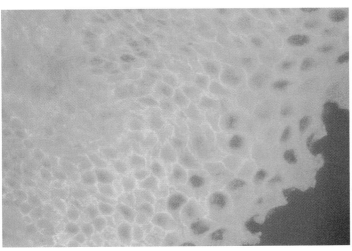

Figure PM-P1-043
Bright yellow immunofluorescence of lgG deposition in a fishnet pattern along the cytoplasmic membranes of epidermal keratinocytes.

Text Links:
U C V 1 **P1-043**
U C V 2 MC-019

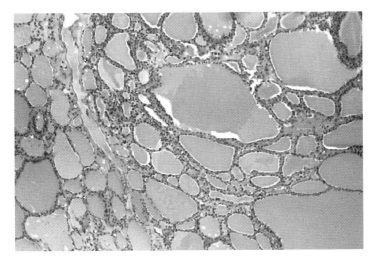

Figure PM-P1-060
Variably sized macrofollicles with abundant colloid.

Text Links:
U C V 1 **P1-060**
U C V 2 MC-094

Figure PM-P1-061
Small hyperchromatic cells with a predominantly papillary architecture invading normal thyroid follicles.

Text Links:
U C V 1 **P1-061**
U C V 2 SUR-008

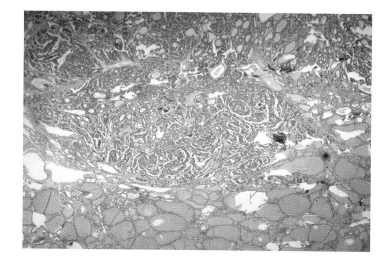

Figure PM-P1-073
Diffuse uniform hyperchromatic cells forming rosettes.

Text Links:
U C V 1 **P1-073**
U C V 2 MC-310

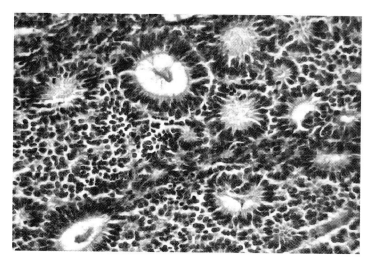

Figure PM-P1-080A
Normal villi with fingerlike projections of columnar epithelium.

Text Links:
U C V 1 **P1-080**
U C V 2 MC-102

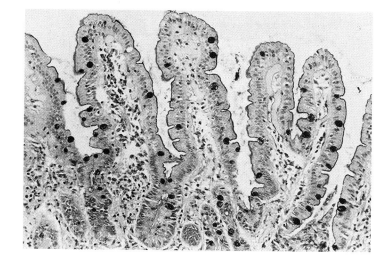

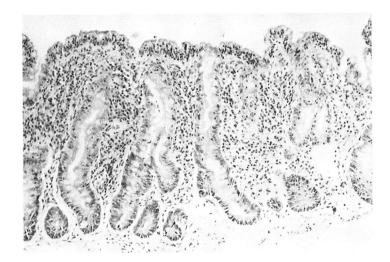

Figure PM-P1-080B
Severe blunting of villi, elongated crypts, and a dense inflammatory infiltrate.

Text Links:
UCV1 **P1-080**
UCV2 MC-102

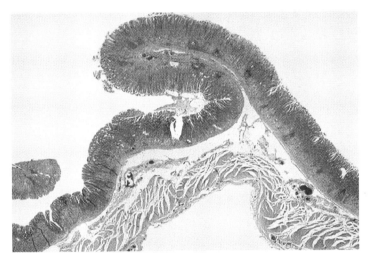

Figure PM-P1-081
Hypercellular gastric mucosa with lymphoid follicles due to dense inflammatory infiltrate in the lamina propia.

Text Links:
UCV1 **P1-081**
UCV2 MC-103

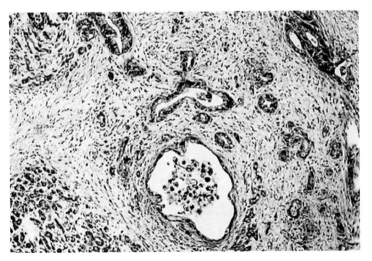

Figure PM-P1-082
Dilated pancreatic ducts, acinar drop out fibrosis, and an inflammatory infiltrate with preservation of the pancreatic islets.

Text Links:
UCV1 **P1-082**
UCV2 IM1-029

Figure PM-P1-086
Colonic mucosa herniating through a defect in the muscularis with adjacent chronic inflammation.

Text Links:
U C V 1 **P1-086**
U C V 2 IM1-031

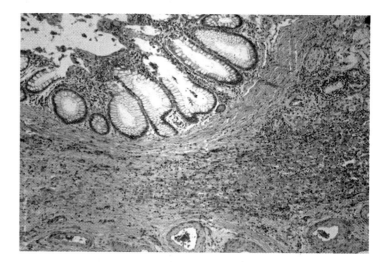

Figure PM-P1-090
Hepatocellular cytoplasmic iron deposition.

Text Links:
U C V 1 **P1-090**
U C V 2 IM1-033

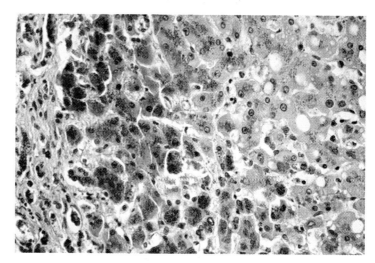

Figure PM-P1-091
Variably sized, regenerating nodules of hepatocytes surrounded by blue staining fibrous bands bridging portal triads.

Text Links:
U C V 1 **P1-091**
U C V 2 IM1-034

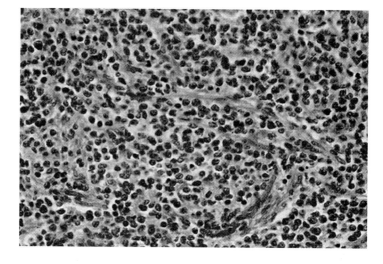

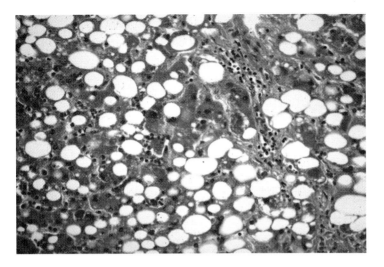

Figure PM-P1-093A
Hepatocytes with
large lipid vacuoles
(macrovesicular
steatosis), neutrophilic
accumulation around
degenerating liver
cells (hepatitis) and
hepatocytes with
eosinophilic cytoplas-
mic inclusions
(Mallory's hyaline).

Text Links:
UCV1 **P1-093**
UCV2 IM1-036

Figure PM-P1-102A
Dense chronic inflam-
matory infiltrate pre-
dominantly limited to
the mucosa with ul-
ceration.

Text Links:
UCV1 **P1-102**
UCV2 IM1-040

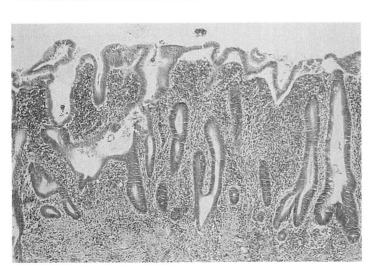

Figure PM-P1-102B
Glandular drop out,
distorted crypts with
blanching, depleted
goblet cells, and a
dense inflammatory
cell infiltrate.

Text Links:
UCV1 **P1-102**
UCV2 IM1-040

Figure PM-P1-103
Pancreatic delta cells
packed with electron
dense membrane
bound granules.

Text Links:
U C V 1 **P1-103**
U C V 2 MC-112

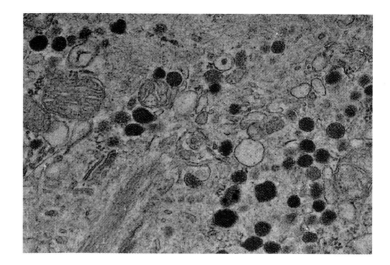

Figure PM-P2-003
Acute inflammation
in the mucosa and ex-
tending into the wall.

Text Links:
U C V 1 **P2-003**
U C V 2 SUR-020

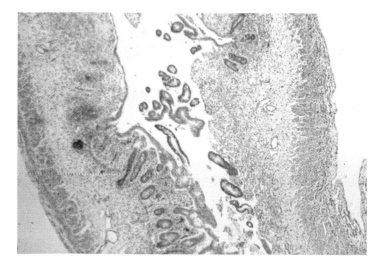

Figure PM-P2-036
Congestion of hepatic
sinusoids by crescent-
shaped erythrocytes.

Text Links:
U C V 1 **P2-036**
U C V 2 PED-021

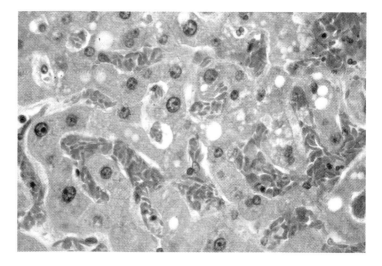

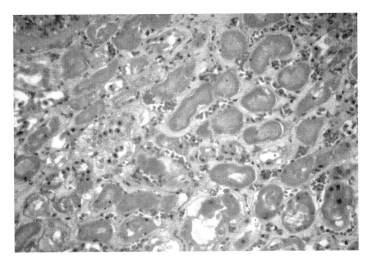

Figure PM-P2-048
Necrosis of tubular epithelial cells lacking nuclei with sloughing into the tubular lumen.

Text Links:
U C V 1 **P2-048**
U C V 2 IM2-032

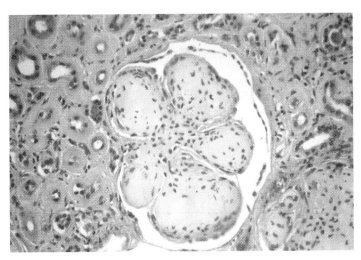

Figure PM-P2-051
Acellular, eosinophilic deposits within the glomerular mesangium.

Text Links:
U C V 1 **P2-051**
U C V 2 MC-197

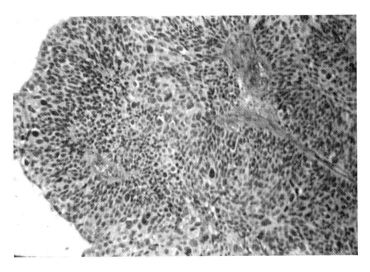

Figure PM-P2-053
Slender papillae lined by multi-layered transitional cells with hyperchromatic, pleomorphic nuclei.

Text Links:
U C V 1 **P2-053**
U C V 2 SUR-036

Figure PM-P2-055
Thickened capillary basement membrane, increased mesangial matrix with eosinophilic nodules; hyaline arteriolosclerosis of the afferent and efferent arterioles (not seen).

Text Links:
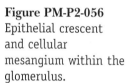 P2-055
UCV2 MC-198

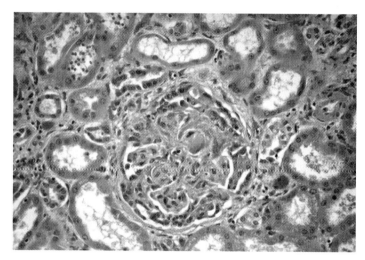

Figure PM-P2-056
Epithelial crescent and cellular mesangium within the glomerulus.

Text Links:
UCV1 P2-056
UCV2 MC-199

Figure PM-P2-062
Normal glomeruli and tubules.

Text Links:
UCV1 P2-062
UCV2 IM2-036

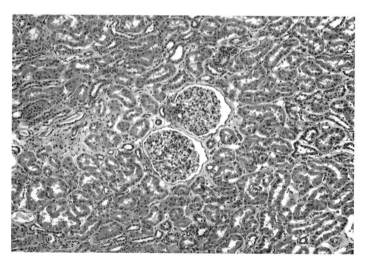

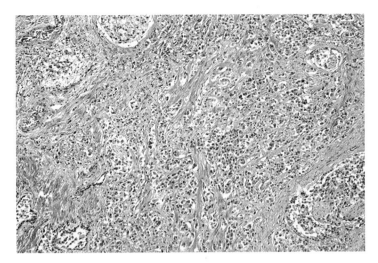

Figure PM-P2-063
Hyperchromatic pleomorphic cells diffusely infiltrating prostatic stroma with focal gland formation and perineural invasion.

Text Links:
UCV1 **P2-063**
UCV2 SUR-037

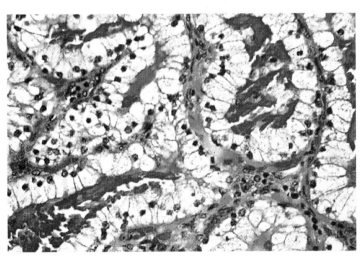

Figure PM-P2-064
Blood filled tubules lined by large polygonal cells with clear cytoplasm.

Text Links:
UCV1 **P2-064**
UCV2 SUR-038

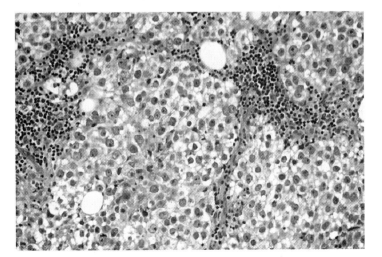

Figure PM-P2-067
Solid nests of germ cells surrounded by fibrous stroma containing lymphocytes.

Text Links:
UCV1 **P2-067**
UCV2 SUR-039

Figure PM-P2-074
Alveolar spaces containing edematous fluid and lined by eosinophilic hyaline membranes and interstitial inflammatory infiltrate.

Text Links:
UCV1 **P2-074**
UCV2 IM2-042

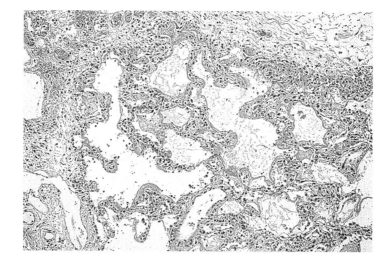

Figure PM-P2-081B
Thin or absent alveolar septa with enlarged airspaces.

Text Links:
UCV1 **P2-081**
UCV2 IM2-046

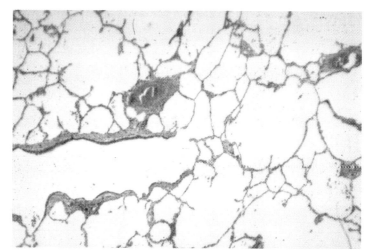

Figure PM-P2-082
Fat globules evident as empty circular spaces within a small pulmonary vessel.

Text Links:
UCV1 **P2-082**
UCV2 MC-063

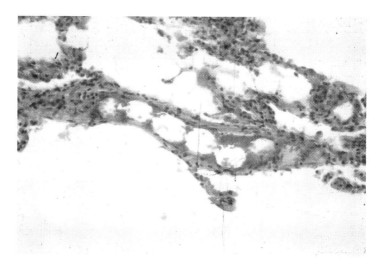

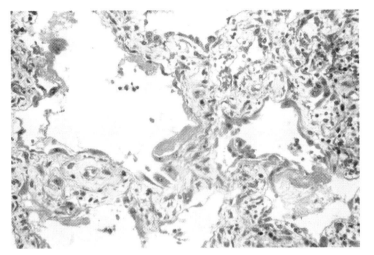

Figure PM-P2-084
Thickened alveolar septa with chronic inflammation and developing interstitial fibrosis.

Text Link:
UCV1 **P2-084**

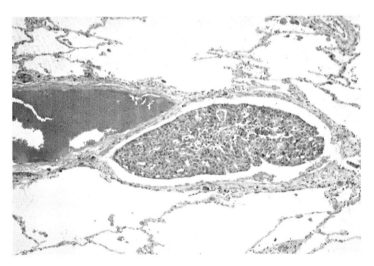

Figure PM-P2-085
Cohesive cellular aggregate of pleomorphic epithelial cells in a lymphatic vessel.

Text Links:
UCV1 **P2-085**
UCV2 SUR-050

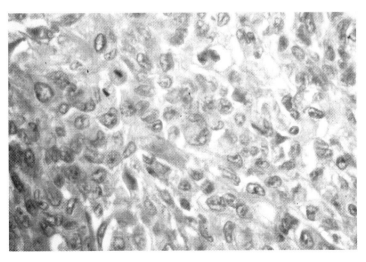

Figure PM-P2-086
Diffuse sheet of epitheloid cells with convoluted, pleomorphic nuclei and mitotic figures.

Text Link:
UCV1 **P2-086**

Figure PM-P2-091
Large thrombus
within the pulmonary
artery.

Text Links:
U C V 1 **P2-091**
U C V 2 ER-046

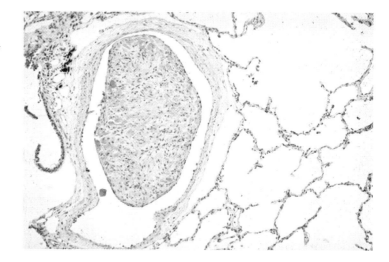

Figure PM-P2-092
Non-caseating granu-
loma composed of
epitheloid histocytes,
multinucleated giant
cells and lymphocytes.

Text Links:
U C V 1 **P2-092**
U C V 2 IM2-048

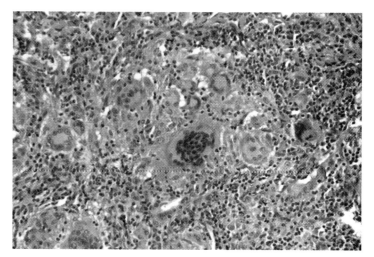

Figure PM-P2-093
Polarized light
microscopy showing
birefringent silica par-
ticles and pigmented
dust with interstitial
fibrosis of the lung.

Text Links:
U C V 1 **P2-093**
U C V 2 IM2-049

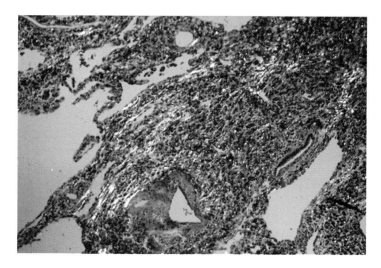

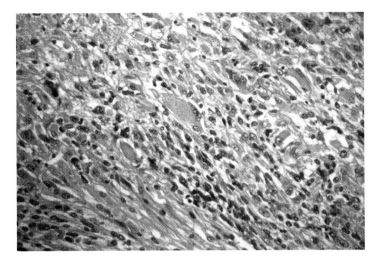

Figure PM-P3-012
Anaplastic cells with areas of focal necrosis and pink, fibrillar cytoplasm.

Text Links:
UCV1 **P3-012**
UCV2 NEU-019

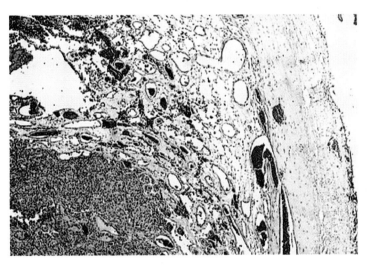

Figure PM-P3-020
Circumscribed region of bland meningothelial cells with whorled pattern and adjacent meninges.

Text Links:
UCV1 **P3-020**
UCV2 MC-249

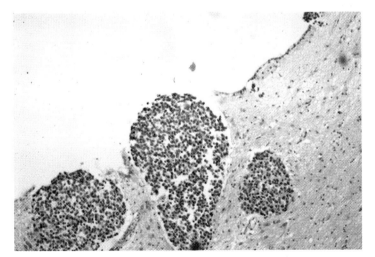

Figure PM-P3-021
Sharply demarcated clusters of cells containing small dark nuclei with scant cytoplasm.

Text Links:
UCV1 **P3-021**
UCV2 MC-252

Figure PM-P3-026
Small primitive cells with hypochromatic nuclei and scant cytoplasm arranged in sheets.

Text Links:
UCV1 **P3-026**
UCV2 NEU-032

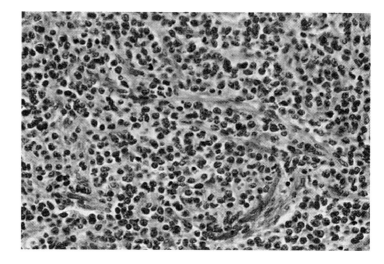

Figure PM-P3-034
Granulomatous inflammation of the media with numerous multinucleated giant cells along degenerated internal elastic lamina. Intimal fibrosis with luminal narrowing.

Text Links:
UCV1 **P3-034**
UCV2 NEU-047

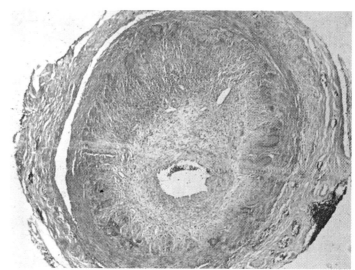

Figure PM-P3-036
Cellular stroma with high mitotic rate and epithelial lined leaf-like architecture.

Text Links:
UCV1 **P3-036**
UCV2 MC-273

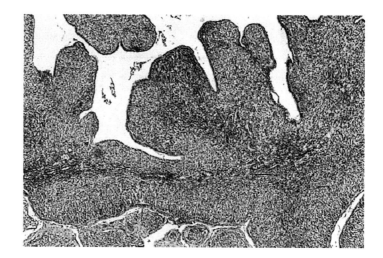

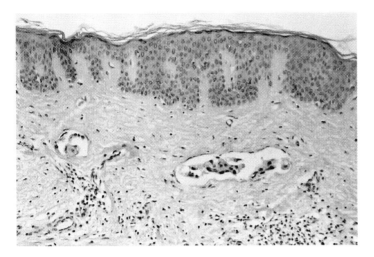

Figure PM-P3-039
Nodules of breast epithelium surrounded by necrotic adipose tissue with an infiltration of macrophages.

Text Link:
U C V 1   P3-039

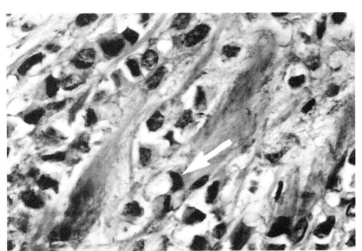

Figure PM-P3-041
Single-file arrangement of cells with pleomorphic nuclei within a fibrous stroma; presence of a signet ring cell.

Text Link:
U C V 1   P3-041

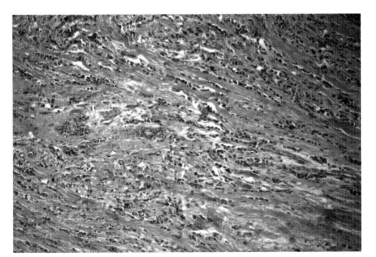

Figure PM-P3-043
Large, poorly differentiated cells arranged in cords infiltrating a dense fibrous stroma.

Text Links:
U C V 1   P3-043
U C V 2   OB-003

Figure PM-P3-044
Elongating, branching glands with bland proliferative epithelium and loose pale fibrous stroma.

Text Links:
UCV1 P3-044
UCV2 MC-277

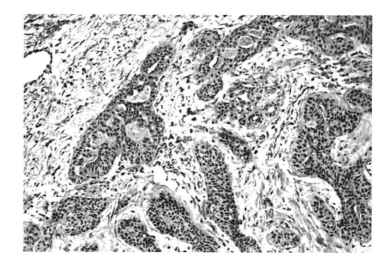

Figure PM-P3-045
Pap smear showing small cells with hyperchromatic nuclei irregular nuclear contours and scant cytoplasm.

Text Link:
UCV1 P3-045

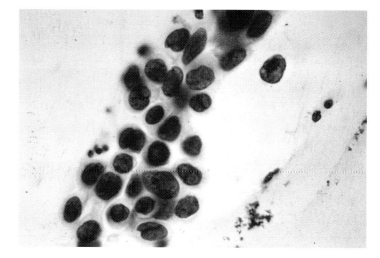

Figure PM-P3-046
Multinucleated syncytiotrophoblasts with vacuolated cytoplasm adjacent to sheet of smaller mononuclear cytotrophoblasts.

Text Links:
UCV1 P3-046
UCV2 OB-006

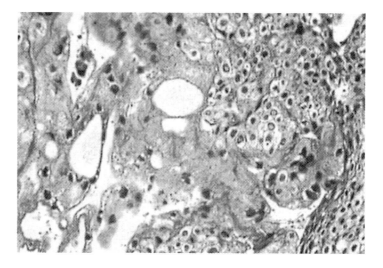

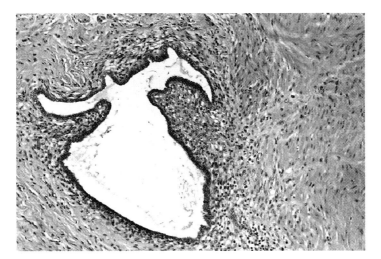

Figure PM-P3-050
Island of ectopic endometrial gland and stroma within the wall of the urinary bladder.

Text Links:
U C V 1 **P3-050**
U C V 2 OB-010

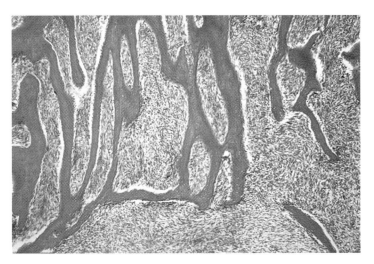

Figure PM-P3-074
Spindle cell proliferation forming abnormal bony trabeculae.

Text Links:
U C V 1 **P3-074**
U C V 2 SUR-045

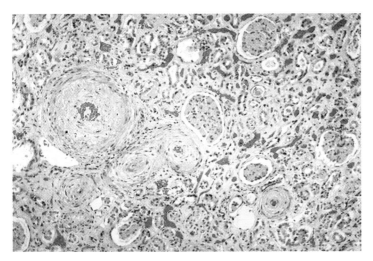

Figure PM-P3-089
Intimal thickening and concentric fibrosis of arterioles in the kidney.

Text Links:
U C V 1 **P3-089**
U C V 2 MC-226

Figure PM-P3-090
Positively birefringent rectangular pleomorphic crystals.

Text Links:
UCV1 **P3-090**
UCV2 MC-380

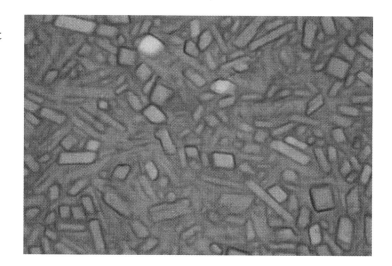

Figure PM-P3-095
Skin biopsy showing a bright green immunofluorescence at the site of IgM deposition along the basement membrane.

Text Links:
UCV1 **P3-095**
UCV2 IM2-056

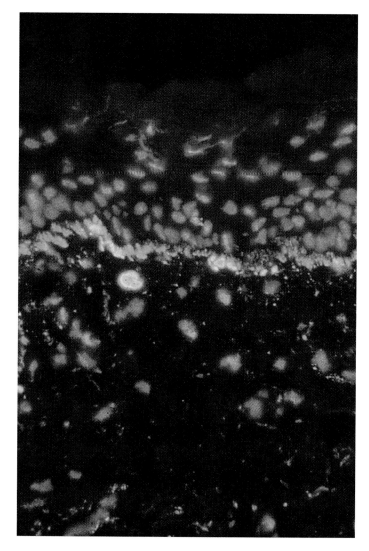

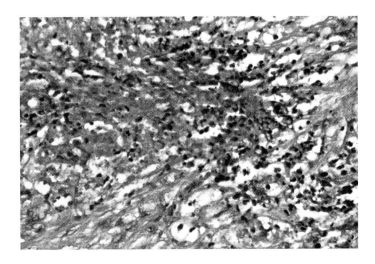

Figure PM-P3-096
"Flea bite" necrosis/microabscesses with neutrophils in the lung; granulomatous formation in the lung parenchyma (not shown).

Text Links:
⬜©Ⓥ① **P3-096**
⬜©Ⓥ② IM2-057

MASTER CASE INDEX

	Case Name	SER	BOOK	SubSpecialty	Case Number
	α₁-Antitrypsin Deficiency	MC	IM-2	Pulmonary	216
	17-Alpha-Hydroxylase Deficiency	UCV-1	BIOCHEM	Endocrinology	1
	17-Alpha-Hydroxylase Deficiency	MC	PED	Endocrinology	304
	5-Alpha-Reductase Deficiency	UCV-1	BIOCHEM	Endocrinology	2
	5-Alpha-Reductase Deficiency	MC	PED	Endocrinology	305
A	Abdominal Aortic Aneurysm	UCV-1	PATHOPHYS-2	General Surgery	1
	Abdominal Aortic Aneurysm	UCV-2	ER	General Surgery	15
	Abdominal Aortic Aneurysm—Ruptured	UCV-1	ANAT	General Surgery	24
	Abortion—Completed	MC	OB/GYN	Obstetrics	287
	Abortion—Incomplete	MC	OB/GYN	Obstetrics	288
	Abortion—Missed	MC	OB/GYN	Obstetrics	289
	Abortion—Spontaneous	UCV-2	OB/GYN	Obstetrics	33
	Abortion—Threatened	UCV-2	ER	Obstetrics	38
	Acetaminophen Overdose	UCV-1	PHARM	Toxicology	92
	Achalasia	UCV-1	PATHOPHYS-1	Gastroenterology	75
	Achalasia	UCV-2	SURG	Gastroenterology	10
	Acne Vulgaris	MC	IM-2	Dermatology	131
	Acoustic Neuroma	MC	SURG	Neurology	368
	Acoustic Schwannoma	UCV-1	ANAT	Neurology	49
	Acromegaly	MC	IM-1	Endocrinology	84
	Acromegaly	UCV-1	BIOCHEM	Endocrinology	3
	Acting Out	UCV-1	BEHAV-SC	Defense Mechanism	13
	Actinic Keratosis	UCV-1	PATHOPHYS-1	Dermatology	29
	Actinic Keratosis	UCV-2	IM-2	Dermatology	3
	Actinomycosis	MC	IM-2	Infectious Disease	157
	Actinomycosis	UCV-1	MICRO-1	Infectious Disease	50
	Acute Adrenal Crisis	UCV-2	ER	Endocrinology	8
	Acute Angle-Closure Glaucoma	UCV-1	PATHOPHYS-1	ENT/Ophthalmology	62
	Acute Angle-Closure Glaucoma	UCV-2	ER	ENT/Ophthalmology	10
	Acute Bacterial Endocarditis	UCV-1	MICRO-1	Cardiology	1
	Acute Bacterial Endocarditis	UCV-2	IM-2	Cardiology	1
	Acute Bronchiolitis	UCV-1	MICRO-1	Infectious Disease	51
	Acute Bronchiolitis	UCV-2	PED	Infectious Disease	24
	Acute Cholecystitis	UCV-1	PATHOPHYS-2	General Surgery	2
	Acute Cholecystitis	UCV-2	SURG	General Surgery	17

Case Name	SER	BOOK	SubSpecialty	Case Number
Acute Conjunctivitis	UCV-1	MICRO-1	ENT/Ophthalmology	17
Acute Cystitis	UCV-1	MICRO-2	Nephrology/Urology	80
Acute Fatty Liver of Pregnancy	MC	OB/GYN	Obstetrics	290
Acute Intermittent Porphyria	MC	ER	Genetics	54
Acute Intermittent Porphyria	UCV-1	BIOCHEM	Genetics	42
Acute Lymphocytic Leukemia (ALL)	UCV-1	PATHOPHYS-2	Hematology/Oncology	13
Acute Lymphocytic Leukemia (ALL)	UCV-2	PED	Hematology/Oncology	16
Acute Myelogenous Leukemia (AML)	UCV-1	PATHOPHYS-2	Hematology/Oncology	14
Acute Myelogenous Leukemia (AML)	UCV-2	IM-1	Hematology/Oncology	41
Acute Renal Failure—Prerenal	MC	ER	Nephrology/Urology	59
Acute Rheumatic Fever	UCV-1	MICRO-1	Infectious Disease	52
Acute Rheumatic Fever	UCV-2	PED	Infectious Disease	25
Acute Sinusitis	MC	ER	ENT/Ophthalmology	29
Acute Sinusitis	UCV-1	MICRO-1	ENT/Ophthalmology	18
Acute Torticollis	UCV-1	ANAT	Neurology	50
Acute Tubular Necrosis—Ischemic	UCV-2	IM-2	Nephrology/Urology	32
Acute Tubular Necrosis—Toxic	UCV-2	IM-2	Nephrology/Urology	33
Acute Tubular Necrosis (ATN)	UCV-1	PATHOPHYS-2	Nephrology/Urology	48
Addison's Disease	UCV-1	BIOCHEM	Endocrinology	4
Addison's Disease	UCV-2	IM-1	Endocrinology	16
Adjustment Disorder	UCV-1	BEHAV-SC	Adjustment Disorders	26
Adjustment Disorder	UCV-2	PSYCH	Adjustment Disorders	4
Adnexal Torsion	MC	OB/GYN	Gynecology	272
Adult Polycystic Kidney Disease	MC	IM-2	Nephrology/Urology	196
Adult Polycystic Kidney Disease (APKD)	UCV-1	PATHOPHYS-2	Nephrology/Urology	49
Adult Respiratory Distress Syndrome (ARDS)	UCV-1	PATHOPHYS-2	Pulmonary	74
Adult Respiratory Distress Syndrome (ARDS)	UCV-2	IM-2	Pulmonary	42
Advance Directives	UCV-2	PSYCH	Ethics	29
Aflatoxin Carcinogenicity	UCV-1	PHARM	Toxicology	93
African Trypanosomiasis	UCV-1	MICRO-1	Infectious Disease	53
Agoraphobia	UCV-2	PSYCH	Anxiety Disorders	5
AIDS—Pediatric	UCV-2	PED	Infectious Disease	26
AIDS Dementia	UCV-1	BEHAV-SC	Neurology	1
AIDS-Related Complex (ARC)	UCV-1	MICRO-1	Infectious Disease	54
Albinism	UCV-1	BIOCHEM	Genetics	43
Alcohol Intoxication	MC	IM-2	Psychopharmacology	206

Case Name	SER	BOOK	SubSpecialty	Case Number
Boerhaave's Syndrome	UCV-1	ANAT	Gastroenterology	15
Borderline Personality Disorder	UCV-1	BEHAV-SC	Personality Disorders	68
Borderline Personality Disorder	UCV-2	PSYCH	Personality Disorders	45
Botulism	UCV-1	MICRO-1	Infectious Disease	66
Botulism	UCV-2	IM-2	Infectious Disease	14
Botulism—Infant	UCV-2	PED	Infectious Disease	27
Brain Abscess	MC	NEURO	Neurology	234
Brain Abscess	UCV-1	MICRO-2	Neurology	87
Breast—Cystosarcoma Phyllodes	MC	OB/GYN	Gynecology	273
Breast—Cystosarcoma Phyllodes	UCV-1	PATHOPHYS-3	Gynecology	36
Breast—Fat Necrosis	UCV-1	PATHOPHYS-3	Gynecology	37
Breast—Fibrocystic Disease	MC	OB/GYN	Gynecology	274
Breast—Fibrocystic Disease	UCV-1	PATHOPHYS-3	Gynecology	38
Breast—Inflammatory Carcinoma	UCV-1	PATHOPHYS-3	Gynecology	39
Breast—Intraductal Papilloma	UCV-1	PATHOPHYS-3	Gynecology	40
Breast—Intraductal Papilloma	UCV-2	OB/GYN	Gynecology	2
Breast—Lobular Carcinoma	UCV-1	PATHOPHYS-3	Gynecology	41
Breast—Paget's Disease	MC	OB/GYN	Gynecology	275
Breast—Paget's Disease	UCV-1	PATHOPHYS-3	Gynecology	42
Breast Abscess	MC	OB/GYN	Gynecology	276
Breast Abscess	UCV-1	MICRO-2	Gynecology	102
Breast Carcinoma	UCV-1	PATHOPHYS-3	Gynecology	43
Breast Carcinoma	UCV-2	OB/GYN	Gynecology	3
Breast Fibroadenoma	MC	OB/GYN	Gynecology	277
Breast Fibroadenoma	UCV-1	PATHOPHYS-3	Gynecology	44
Brief Psychotic Disorder	UCV-2	PSYCH	Psychotic Disorders	47
Brief Psychotic Episode	UCV-1	BEHAV-SC	Psychotic Disorders	77
Bronchiectasis	MC	IM-2	Pulmonary	208
Bronchiectasis	UCV-1	PATHOPHYS-2	Pulmonary	78
Brown-Séquard Syndrome	UCV-1	ANAT	Neurology	54
Brown-Séquard Syndrome	UCV-2	NEURO	Neurology	4
Brucellosis	MC	IM-2	Infectious Disease	162
Brucellosis	UCV-1	MICRO-1	Infectious Disease	67
Bruton's Agammaglobulinemia	UCV-2	PED	Immunology	36
Budd–Chiari Syndrome	MC	IM-1	Gastroenterology	99
Budd–Chiari Syndrome	UCV-1	PATHOPHYS-1	Gastroenterology	78
Bulimia Nervosa	UCV-1	BEHAV-SC	Eating Disorders	46
Bulimia Nervosa	UCV-2	PSYCH	Eating Disorders	28

Case Name	SER	BOOK	SubSpecialty	Case Number
Bullous Pemphigoid	MC	ER	Dermatology	17
Burkitt's Lymphoma	UCV-1	PATHOPHYS-2	Hematology/Oncology	18
Burkitt's Lymphoma	UCV-2	IM-1	Hematology/Oncology	44
C				
C1 Spinal Cord Injury	UCV-1	PATHOPHYS-3	Neurology	3
CAD—Myocardial Infarction	UCV-1	PATHOPHYS-1	Cardiology	7
CAD—Myocardial Infarction	UCV-2	ER	Cardiology	2
CAD—Prinzmetal's Angina	MC	ER	Cardiology	2
CAD—Unstable Angina	MC	ER	Cardiology	3
Caffeine Intoxication	UCV-1	PHARM	Psychopharmacology	75
Campylobacter Enteritis	UCV-1	MICRO-1	Infectious Disease	68
Candida Esophagitis	MC	IM-1	Gastroenterology	100
Candida Esophagitis	UCV-1	PATHOPHYS-1	Gastroenterology	79
Candidiasis	UCV-1	MICRO-1	Infectious Disease	69
Cannabis Intoxication	UCV-1	PHARM	Psychopharmacology	76
Cannabis Intoxication	UCV-2	PSYCH	Psychopharmacology	18
Captopril Side Effects	UCV-1	PHARM	Cardiology	3
Caput Succedaneum	UCV-1	ANAT	Neonatology	43
Carbamazepine Side Effects	UCV-1	PHARM	Neurology	64
Carbamazepine Toxicity	MC	NEURO	Neurology	235
Carbon Dioxide Narcosis	UCV-1	PATHOPHYS-3	Toxicology	97
Carbon Monoxide Poisoning	UCV-1	BIOCHEM	Pulmonary	95
Carbon Monoxide Poisoning	UCV-2	ER	Toxicology	47
Carcinoid Syndrome	MC	IM-1	Gastroenterology	101
Carcinoid Syndrome	UCV-1	BIOCHEM	Gastroenterology	37
Cardiac Tamponade	UCV-1	ANAT	Cardiology	3
Cardiac Tamponade	UCV-1	PATHOPHYS-1	Cardiology	8
Cardiac Tamponade	UCV-2	ER	Cardiology	3
Cardiac Transplant	UCV-1	PATHOPHYS-1	Cardiology	9
Cat-Scratch Disease	UCV-1	MICRO-1	Infectious Disease	70
Cauda Equina Syndrome	MC	NEURO	Neurology	236
Cauda Equina Syndrome	UCV-1	PATHOPHYS-3	Neurology	4
Caustic Ingestion	MC	ER	Toxicology	66
Cavernous Sinus Thrombosis	MC	NEURO	Neurology	237
Cavernous Sinus Thrombosis	UCV-1	ANAT	Neurology	55
Cecal Carcinoma	UCV-1	PATHOPHYS-2	General Surgery	4
Celiac Disease	MC	IM-1	Gastroenterology	102
Celiac Disease	UCV-1	PATHOPHYS-1	Gastroenterology	80
Cellulitis	MC	IM-2	Dermatology	133

Case Name	SER	BOOK	SubSpecialty	Case Number
Cellulitis	UCV-1	MICRO-1	Dermatology	6
Cerebellopontine Angle Compression	MC	NEURO	Neurology	238
Cerebral Aneurysm	MC	NEURO	Neurology	239
Cerebral Aneurysm	UCV-1	PATHOPHYS-3	Neurology	5
Cerebral Palsy	UCV-2	NEURO	Neurology	5
Cervical Carcinoma	UCV-2	OB/GYN	Gynecology	4
Cervical Carcinoma (In Situ)	UCV-1	PATHOPHYS-3	Gynecology	45
Cervical Polyps	MC	OB/GYN	Gynecology	278
Cervicitis	MC	OB/GYN	Gynecology	279
Chagas' Disease	MC	IM-2	Infectious Disease	163
Chagas' Disease	UCV-1	MICRO-1	Infectious Disease	71
Chalazion	MC	ER	ENT/Ophthalmology	38
Chancroid	UCV-2	OB/GYN	Gynecology	5
Chédiak–Higashi Syndrome	MC	IM-2	Genetics	154
Chédiak–Higashi Syndrome	UCV-1	MICRO-1	Genetics	45
Child Abuse—Physical	UCV-2	PED	Psychiatry—Child	53
Child Abuse—Sexual	UCV-2	PSYCH	Child	13
Child Abuse—Shaken Baby Syndrome	UCV-1	BEHAV-SC	Child Psychiatry	34
Chlamydia Pneumonia	MC	IM-2	Infectious Disease	164
Chlamydia Pneumonia	UCV-1	MICRO-1	Infectious Disease	72
Chlamydia trachomatis	UCV-1	MICRO-1	Infectious Disease	73
Chloramphenicol Side Effects	UCV-1	PHARM	Infectious Disease	46
Chloroquine Toxicity	UCV-1	PHARM	Infectious Disease	47
Choanal Atresia	UCV-1	ANAT	ENT/Ophthalmology	10
Choking	UCV-1	ANAT	ENT/Ophthalmology	11
Cholangiocarcinoma	MC	SURG	General Surgery	343
Choledocholithiasis	MC	SURG	General Surgery	344
Cholelithiasis	MC	SURG	General Surgery	345
Cholera	MC	ER	Infectious Disease	57
Cholera	UCV-1	MICRO-1	Infectious Disease	74
Cholestatic Jaundice of Pregnancy	UCV-2	OB/GYN	Obstetrics	37
Chorioamnionitis	UCV-1	MICRO-2	Obstetrics	107
Chorioamnionitis	UCV-2	OB/GYN	Obstetrics	38
Choriocarcinoma	UCV-1	PATHOPHYS-3	Gynecology	46
Choriocarcinoma	UCV-2	OB/GYN	Gynecology	6
Chronic Atrophic Gastritis	MC	IM-1	Gastroenterology	103
Chronic Atrophic Gastritis	UCV-1	PATHOPHYS-1	Gastroenterology	81
Chronic Granulomatous Disease	MC	PED	Immunology	328

Case Name	SER	BOOK	SubSpecialty	Case Number
Delirium	UCV-2	PSYCH	Neurology	1
Delirium—Inhalant Abuse	UCV-1	BEHAV-SC	Neurology	3
Delirium—Medical Cause	UCV-1	BEHAV-SC	Neurology	4
Delirium Tremens	UCV-2	PSYCH	Psychopharmacology	20
Delusional Disorder	UCV-1	BEHAV-SC	Psychotic Disorders	78
Delusional Disorder	UCV-2	PSYCH	Psychotic Disorders	48
Dementia—Alzheimer's	UCV-2	PSYCH	Neurology	2
Dementia—Alzheimer's	UCV-1	BEHAV-SC	Neurology	5
Dementia—Vascular	UCV-2	NEURO	Neurology	17
Dementia—Vascular	UCV-1	BEHAV-SC	Neurology	6
Denial	UCV-1	BEHAV-SC	Defense Mechanism	14
Dependent Personality Disorder	UCV-1	BEHAV-SC	Personality Disorders	69
Depression—Elderly	UCV-1	BEHAV-SC	Mood Disorders	53
Depression—Suicidal	UCV-2	ER	Psychiatry-Mood Disorders	44
Depression—Suicidal	UCV-1	BEHAV-SC	Mood Disorders	54
Depression—Suicidal	UCV-2	PSYCH	Mood Disorders	41
Depressive Episode—Major	UCV-2	PSYCH	Mood Disorders	42
Depressive Episode—Major	UCV-1	BEHAV-SC	Mood Disorders	55
Dermatitis Herpetiformis	UCV-1	PATHOPHYS-1	Dermatology	33
Dermatitis Herpetiformis	UCV-2	IM-2	Dermatology	5
Dermatomyositis	UCV-1	PATHOPHYS-3	Rheumatology	81
Dermatomyositis	UCV-2	IM-2	Rheumatology	51
Desmoid Tumor	UCV-1	PATHOPHYS-3	Gynecology	47
Devaluation	UCV-1	BEHAV-SC	Defense Mechanism	15
Diabetes in Pregnancy	UCV-2	OB/GYN	Obstetrics	39
Diabetes Insipidus	UCV-1	BIOCHEM	Endocrinology	7
Diabetes Mellitus Type I (Juvenile Onset)	UCV-1	PATHOPHYS-1	Endocrinology	51
Diabetes Mellitus Type I (Juvenile Onset)	UCV-2	IM-1	Endocrinology	18
Diabetes Mellitus Type II (Adult Onset)	MC	IM-1	Endocrinology	88
Diabetes Mellitus Type II (Adult Onset)	UCV-1	PATHOPHYS-1	Endocrinology	52
Diabetic Ketoacidosis	UCV-1	BIOCHEM	Endocrinology	8
Diabetic Ketoacidosis	UCV-2	IM-1	Endocrinology	19
Diabetic Nephropathy	MC	IM-2	Nephrology/Urology	198
Diabetic Nephropathy	UCV-1	PATHOPHYS-2	Nephrology/Urology	55
Diagnosis of Pregnancy	UCV-2	OB/GYN	Obstetrics	40
Diaper Rash	MC	PED	Dermatology	298
Didanosine Toxicity	UCV-1	PHARM	Toxicology	98
Diethylstilbestrol (DES) Exposure	UCV-1	PHARM	Endocrinology	16

F

H

Case Name	SER	BOOK	SubSpecialty	Case Number
Methanol Poisoning	UCV-1	PHARM	Toxicology	103
Methanol Poisoning	UCV-2	ER	Toxicology	48
Methemoglobinemia	MC	IM-1	Hematology/Oncology	125
Methemoglobinemia	UCV-1	BIOCHEM	Hematology/Oncology	81
Methotrexate Toxicity	UCV-1	PHARM	Hematology/Oncology	40
Methyldopa Side Effects	UCV-1	PHARM	Cardiology	6
Methylxanthine Toxicity	MC	ER	Toxicology	71
Migraine	UCV-1	PATHOPHYS-3	Neurology	22
Migraine	UCV-2	NEURO	Neurology	28
Minimal Change Disease	UCV-1	PATHOPHYS-2	Nephrology/Urology	62
Minimal Change Disease	UCV-2	IM-2	Nephrology/Urology	36
Mitral Insufficiency	UCV-1	PATHOPHYS-1	Cardiology	20
Mitral Insufficiency	UCV-2	IM-1	Cardiology	9
Mitral Stenosis	UCV-1	PATHOPHYS-1	Cardiology	21
Mitral Stenosis	UCV-2	IM-1	Cardiology	10
Mittelschmerz	MC	OB/GYN	Gynecology	282
Mixed Connective Tissue Disorder	MC	IM-2	Rheumatology	222
Mixed Connective Tissue Disorder	UCV-1	PATHOPHYS-3	Rheumatology	83
Molluscum Contagiosum	MC	IM-2	Dermatology	143
Molluscum Contagiosum	UCV-1	MICRO-1	Dermatology	11
Monoclonal Gammopathy of Undetermined Significance	MC	IM-1	Hematology/Oncology	126
Mononeuritis Multiplex	MC	NEURO	Neurology	253
Mucormycosis	UCV-1	MICRO-2	Infectious Disease	25
Multifocal Atrial Tachycardia	MC	IM-1	Cardiology	79
Multiple Endocrine Neoplasia (MEN)	MC	IM-1	Endocrinology	93
Multiple Myeloma	UCV-1	PATHOPHYS-2	Hematology/Oncology	31
Multiple Myeloma	UCV-2	IM-1	Hematology/Oncology	50
Multiple Sclerosis	UCV-1	PATHOPHYS-3	Neurology	23
Multiple Sclerosis	UCV-2	NEURO	Neurology	29
Multisystem Organ Failure (MSOF)	MC	ER	Cardiology	10
Mumps	MC	PED	Infectious Disease	325
Mumps	UCV-1	MICRO-2	Infectious Disease	26
Munchausen's Syndrome	UCV-1	BEHAV-SC	Factitious Disorders	48
Mushroom Poisoning	UCV-1	PHARM	Toxicology	104
Myasthenia Gravis	UCV-1	PATHOPHYS-3	Neurology	24
Myasthenia Gravis	UCV-2	NEURO	Neurology	30
Mycoplasma Pneumonia	MC	IM-2	Infectious Disease	182

Case Name	SER	BOOK	SubSpecialty	Case Number
Mycoplasma Pneumonia	UCV-1	MICRO-2	Infectious Disease	27
Mycosis Fungoides	UCV-1	PATHOPHYS-1	Dermatology	41
Mycosis Fungoides—Sézary Syndrome	MC	IM-2	Dermatology	144
Myelodysplastic Syndromes	MC	IM-1	Hematology/Oncology	27
Myelofibrosis with Myeloid Metaplasia	UCV-1	PATHOPHYS-2	Hematology/Oncology	32
Myocarditis	UCV-1	PATHOPHYS-1	Cardiology	22
Myocarditis—Viral	MC	IM-1	Cardiology	80
Myocarditis—Viral	UCV-1	MICRO-1	Cardiology	2
Myotonic Dystrophy	UCV-1	PATHOPHYS-3	Neurology	25
Myotonic Dystrophy	UCV-2	NEURO	Neurology	31
Narcissistic Personality Disorder	UCV-1	BEHAV-SC	Personality Disorders	71
N				
Narcolepsy	MC	NEURO	Neurology	254
Narcolepsy	UCV-1	BEHAV-SC	Neurology	7
Necrotizing Enterocolitis	UCV-1	MICRO-1	Gastroenterology	33
Necrotizing Enterocolitis	UCV-2	PED	Neonatology	43
Necrotizing Fasciitis	UCV-1	MICRO-2	Infectious Disease	28
Neonatal Meningitis	UCV-2	PED	Neonatology	44
Neonatal Sepsis	UCV-2	ER	Neonatology	29
Nephrolithiasis	UCV-1	ANAT	Nephrology/Urology	47
Nephrolithiasis	UCV-2	ER	Nephrology/Urology	30
Nephrotic Syndrome	MC	IM-2	Nephrology/Urology	203
Neuroblastoma	UCV-1	PATHOPHYS-3	Neurology	26
Neuroblastoma	UCV-2	NEURO	Neurology	32
Neurofibromatosis Type 1	MC	NEURO	Neurology	255
Neuroleptic Malignant Syndrome	UCV-1	PHARM	Psychopharmacology	84
Neuroleptic Malignant Syndrome	UCV-2	ER	Psychopharmacology	41
Neurosyphilis (Tabes Dorsalis)	UCV-2	IM-2	Infectious Disease	28
Neutropenic Enterocolitis	UCV-1	MICRO-1	Gastroenterology	34
Nevirapine Therapy	UCV-1	PHARM	Toxicology	105
Niacin Side Effects	UCV-1	PHARM	Cardiology	7
Nicotine Withdrawal	UCV-1	PHARM	Psychopharmacology	85
Niemann–Pick Disease	UCV-1	BIOCHEM	Genetics	65
Nitrate Exposure	UCV-1	PHARM	Cardiology	8
Nitroglycerin Tolerance	UCV-1	PHARM	Cardiology	9
Nocardiosis	UCV-1	MICRO-2	Infectious Disease	29
Non-Hodgkin's Lymphoma	UCV-1	PATHOPHYS-2	Hematology/Oncology	33
Non-Hodgkin's Lymphoma	UCV-2	IM-1	Hematology/Oncology	51
Nonketotic Hyperosmolar Coma	UCV-1	BIOCHEM	Endocrinology	24

O

P

Case Name	SER	BOOK	SubSpecialty	Case Number
Parkinson's Disease	UCV-2	NEURO	Neurology	34
Parkinson's Disease—MPTP-Induced	UCV-1	PHARM	Neurology	69
Parotid Gland—Pleomorphic Adenoma	MC	SURG	General Surgery	357
Paroxysmal Nocturnal Hemoglobinuria	MC	IM-1	Hematology/Oncology	128
Paroxysmal Nocturnal Hemoglobinuria	UCV-1	BIOCHEM	Hematology/Oncology	82
Paroxysmal Supraventricular Tachycardia	UCV-2	IM-1	Cardiology	11
Passive-Aggressive Personality Disorder	UCV-1	BEHAV-SC	Personality Disorders	74
Pasteurella multocida	UCV-1	MICRO-2	Infectious Disease	33
Patent Ductus Arteriosus	UCV-1	ANAT	Cardiology	6
Patent Ductus Arteriosus	UCV-2	PED	Cardiology	1
Patient Autonomy	UCV-2	PSYCH	Ethics	32
Patient-Doctor Confidentiality	UCV-2	PSYCH	Ethics	33
PCP Intoxication	UCV-1	BEHAV-SC	Psychopharmacology	97
PCP Intoxication	UCV-2	PSYCH	Psychopharmacology	25
Pediculosis	MC	IM-2	Dermatology	146
Pedophilia	UCV-1	BEHAV-SC	Paraphilia	63
Pelvic Fracture	MC	SURG	Orthopedics	374
Pelvic Fracture	UCV-1	ANAT	Orthopedics	92
Pelvic Inflammatory Disease	UCV-1	MICRO-2	Gynecology	104
Pelvic Inflammatory Disease	UCV-2	OB/GYN	Gynecology	18
Pelvic Tuberculosis	UCV-1	MICRO-2	Gynecology	105
Pelvic Tuberculosis	UCV-2	OB/GYN	Gynecology	19
Pemphigus	MC	ER	Dermatology	19
Pemphigus	UCV-1	PATHOPHYS-1	Dermatology	43
Penetrating Anterior Abdominal Wound	UCV-2	ER	General Surgery	18
Penetrating Thoracic Injury	UCV-2	ER	General Surgery	19
Penicillin Allergic Reaction	UCV-1	PHARM	Infectious Disease	52
Peptic Ulcer—Perforated	UCV-2	SURG	Gastroenterology	14
Peptic Ulcer—Perforated	UCV-1	ANAT	Gastroenterology	21
Peptic Ulcer Disease	UCV-2	IM-1	Gastroenterology	38
Peptic Ulcer Disease (H pylori)	UCV-1	MICRO-1	Gastroenterology	35
Perianal Abscess	MC	SURG	General Surgery	358
Pericardial Effusion	MC	IM-1	Cardiology	81
Pericarditis—Acute	UCV-2	IM-1	Cardiology	12
Pericarditis—Acute	UCV-1	MICRO-1	Cardiology	3
Peripheral Arterial Embolism	UCV-1	PATHOPHYS-1	Cardiology	23
Peripheral Neuropathy—Diabetic	MC	NEURO	Neurology	259
Peripheral Neuropathy—Diabetic	UCV-1	PATHOPHYS-3	Neurology	29

Case Name	SER	BOOK	SubSpecialty	Case Number
Peripheral Neuropathy due to Vincristine	UCV-2	NEURO	Neurology	35
Peritonsillar Abscess	MC	ER	ENT/Ophthalmology	36
Petit's Triangle Hernia	MC	SURG	General Surgery	359
Petit's Triangle Hernia	UCV-1	ANAT	General Surgery	31
Peutz–Jeghers Syndrome	UCV-1	PATHOPHYS-1	Gastroenterology	98
Pharyngitis—Adenoviral	MC	IM-1	ENT/Ophthalmology	96
Pharyngitis—Adenovirus	UCV-1	MICRO-1	ENT/Ophthalmology	25
Pharyngitis—Streptococcal	MC	IM-1	ENT/Ophthalmology	97
Pharyngitis—Streptococcal	UCV-1	MICRO-1	ENT/Ophthalmology	26
Phenylketonuria (PKU)	UCV-1	BIOCHEM	Genetics	67
Phenylketonuria (PKU)	UCV-2	PED	Genetics	14
Phenytoin Overdose	UCV-1	PHARM	Neurology	70
Pheochromocytoma	UCV-1	BIOCHEM	Endocrinology	26
Pheochromocytoma	UCV-2	SURG	Endocrinology	7
Phosphoenolpyruvate Carboxykinase Deficiency	UCV-1	BIOCHEM	Genetics	68
Physiologic Jaundice Of Newborn	UCV-2	PED	Neonatology	45
Pick's Disease	UCV-2	NEURO	Neurology	36
Pilonidal Cyst	MC	SURG	General Surgery	360
Pinealoma	UCV-1	PATHOPHYS-1	Endocrinology	58
Pinworm Infection	UCV-1	MICRO-1	Gastroenterology	36
Pityriasis Alba	MC	PED	Dermatology	301
Pityriasis Rosea	MC	IM-2	Dermatology	147
Pityriasis Rosea	UCV-1	PATHOPHYS-1	Dermatology	44
Pityriasis Versicolor	MC	IM-2	Dermatology	148
Pityriasis Versicolor	UCV-1	MICRO-1	Dermatology	12
Placenta Previa	UCV-2	OB/GYN	Obstetrics	43
Placental Abruption	UCV-2	OB/GYN	Obstetrics	44
Plague	UCV-1	MICRO-2	Infectious Disease	34
Pleural Effusion	UCV-1	PATHOPHYS-2	Pulmonary	87
Plummer–Vinson Syndrome	UCV-1	PATHOPHYS-1	Gastroenterology	99
Plummer–Vinson Syndrome	UCV-2	SURG	Gastroenterology	15
Pneumococcal Pneumonia	UCV-1	MICRO-2	Infectious Disease	35
Pneumococcal Pneumonia	UCV-2	IM-2	Infectious Disease	25
Pneumocystis carinii Pneumonia	UCV-1	MICRO-2	Infectious Disease	36
Pneumothorax—Open	MC	ER	Pulmonary	65
Pneumothorax—Spontaneous	UCV-2	IM-2	Pulmonary	47
Pneumothorax—Spontaneous	UCV-1	PATHOPHYS-2	Pulmonary	88
Pneumothorax—Tension	UCV-2	SURG	Pulmonary	51

Case Name	SER	BOOK	SubSpecialty	Case Number
Pneumothorax—Tension	UCV-1	PATHOPHYS-2	Pulmonary	89
Poliomyelitis	UCV-1	MICRO-2	Neurology	96
Poliomyelitis	UCV-2	NEURO	Neurology	37
Polyarteritis Nodosa	UCV-1	PATHOPHYS-3	Rheumatology	86
Polyarteritis Nodosa	UCV-2	IM-2	Rheumatology	53
Polycystic Ovary Disease	UCV-1	PATHOPHYS-3	Gynecology	56
Polycystic Ovary Disease	UCV-2	OB/GYN	Gynecology	20
Polycythemia Vera (PCV)	UCV-1	PATHOPHYS-2	Hematology/Oncology	34
Polycythemia Vera (PCV)	UCV-2	IM-1	Hematology/Oncology	52
Polyhydramnios	UCV-2	OB/GYN	Obstetrics	45
Polymyalgia Rheumatica	MC	IM-2	Rheumatology	224
Polymyalgia Rheumatica	UCV-1	PATHOPHYS-3	Rheumatology	87
Polymyositis	MC	IM-2	Rheumatology	225
Polymyositis	UCV-1	PATHOPHYS-3	Rheumatology	88
Pompe's Disease	UCV-1	BIOCHEM	Genetics	69
Popliteal Fossa Trauma	UCV-1	ANAT	General Surgery	32
Porphyria Cutanea Tarda	MC	IM-2	Genetics	156
Porphyria Cutanea Tarda	UCV-1	BIOCHEM	Genetics	70
Portal Hypertension	UCV-1	ANAT	Gastroenterology	22
Portal Hypertension	UCV-2	SURG	Gastroenterology	16
Portal Vein Thrombosis	UCV-2	PED	Gastroenterology	8
Port-Wine Stain	MC	SURG	Dermatology	337
Postpartum Hemorrhage	MC	OB/GYN	Obstetrics	295
Postpartum Hemorrhage	UCV-1	PATHOPHYS-3	Obstetrics	64
Postpartum Thrombophlebitis	UCV-1	PATHOPHYS-3	Obstetrics	65
Poststreptococcal Glomerulonephritis	UCV-1	MICRO-2	Nephrology/Urology	83
Poststreptococcal Glomerulonephritis	UCV-2	PED	Nephrology/Urology	47
Post-Traumatic Stress Disorder	UCV-1	BEHAV-SC	Anxiety Disorders	30
Post-Traumatic Stress Disorder	UCV-2	PSYCH	Anxiety Disorders	9
Post-Traumatic Stress Disorder (Child)	UCV-1	BEHAV-SC	Child Psychiatry	37
Precocious Puberty	MC	PED	Endocrinology	307
Precocious Puberty	UCV-1	BIOCHEM	Endocrinology	27
Pregnancy with IUD	UCV-2	OB/GYN	Obstetrics	46
Premenstrual Dysphoric Disorder	UCV-1	BEHAV-SC	Mood Disorders	59
Premenstrual Dysphoric Disorder	UCV-2	OB/GYN	Gynecology	21
Presbycusis	UCV-1	PATHOPHYS-1	ENT/Ophthalmology	69
Presbyopia	UCV-1	PATHOPHYS-1	ENT/Ophthalmology	70
Primary Amenorrhea—Testicular Feminization	UCV-1	BIOCHEM	Gynecology	87

Case Name	SER	BOOK	SubSpecialty	Case Number
Primary Amenorrhea—Testicular Feminization	UCV-2	OB/GYN	Gynecology	22
Primary Amenorrhea—Turner's Syndrome	UCV-1	PATHOPHYS-3	Gynecology	57
Primary Amenorrhea—Turner's Syndrome	UCV-2	OB/GYN	Gynecology	23
Primary Biliary Cirrhosis	UCV-1	PATHOPHYS-1	Gastroenterology	100
Primary Biliary Cirrhosis	UCV-2	IM-1	Gastroenterology	39
Primary Insomnia	UCV-1	BEHAV-SC	Sleep Disorders	86
Primary Pulmonary Hypertension	MC	IM-2	Pulmonary	214
Primary Pulmonary Hypertension	UCV-1	PATHOPHYS-2	Pulmonary	90
Primary Sclerosing Cholangitis	MC	IM-1	Gastroenterology	109
Proctocolitis	MC	IM-2	Infectious Disease	183
Proctocolitis	UCV-1	MICRO-2	Infectious Disease	37
Progressive Multifocal Leukoencephalopathy	MC	NEURO	Neurology	260
Progressive Multifocal Leukoencephalopathy	UCV-1	MICRO-2	Neurology	97
Progressive Systemic Sclerosis (Scleroderma)	MC	IM-2	Rheumatology	226
Progressive Systemic Sclerosis (Scleroderma)	UCV-1	PATHOPHYS-3	Rheumatology	89
Prolactinoma	UCV-1	PATHOPHYS-1	Endocrinology	59
Prostate Carcinoma	UCV-1	PATHOPHYS-2	Nephrology/Urology	63
Prostate Carcinoma	UCV-2	SURG	Nephrology/Urology	37
Prostatitis—Acute	UCV-1	MICRO-2	Nephrology/Urology	84
Prostatitis—Chronic	UCV-1	MICRO-2	Nephrology/Urology	85
Prosthetic Valve Endocarditis	MC	ER	Cardiology	11
Prosthetic Valve Endocarditis	UCV-1	MICRO-1	Cardiology	4
Protease Inhibitor Side Effects	UCV-1	PHARM	Toxicology	109
Pseudobulbar Palsy	MC	NEURO	Neurology	261
Pseudobulbar Palsy	UCV-1	PATHOPHYS-3	Neurology	30
Pseudocyesis	UCV-1	BEHAV-SC	Somatoform Disorders	92
Pseudodementia	MC	NEURO	Psychiatry-Mood Disorders	269
Pseudogout	MC	SURG	Rheumatology	380
Pseudogout	UCV-1	PATHOPHYS-3	Rheumatology	90
Pseudohyperkalemia	MC	ER	Endocrinology	26
Pseudohypoparathyroidism	UCV-1	BIOCHEM	Endocrinology	28
Pseudomembranous Colitis	MC	IM-1	Gastroenterology	110
Pseudomembranous Colitis	UCV-1	PHARM	Gastroenterology	31
Pseudoseizures	MC	NEURO	Psychiatry-Factitious Disorders	268
Pseudotumor Cerebri	UCV-1	PATHOPHYS-1	ENT/Ophthalmology	71
Pseudotumor Cerebri	UCV-2	NEURO	Neurology	38
Psittacosis	UCV-1	MICRO-2	Infectious Disease	38
Psoriasis	UCV-1	PATHOPHYS-1	Dermatology	45

Case Name	SER	BOOK	SubSpecialty	Case Number
Seizure, Grand Mal	UCV-2	NEURO	Neurology	43
Seizure, Jacksonian Type	UCV-1	BEHAV-SC	Neurology	10
Seizure, Metastatic Disease	UCV-2	NEURO	Neurology	44
Seizure, Temporal Lobe	UCV-1	BEHAV-SC	Neurology	11
Selective IgA Deficiency	UCV-1	MICRO-2	Immunology	4
Seminoma	UCV-1	PATHOPHYS-2	Nephrology/Urology	67
Seminoma	UCV-2	SURG	Nephrology/Urology	39
Separation Anxiety	UCV-1	BEHAV-SC	Child Psychiatry	38
Septic Arthritis—Gonococcal	UCV-1	MICRO-2	Orthopedics	110
Septic Arthritis—Staphylococcal	UCV-1	PATHOPHYS-3	Orthopedics	76
Septic Arthritis—Staphylococcal	UCV-2	IM-2	Orthopedics	41
Serum Sickness	UCV-1	PATHOPHYS-2	Immunology	44
Severe Combined Immunodeficiency (SCID)	UCV-1	MICRO-2	Immunology	5
Severe Combined Immunodeficiency	UCV-2	PED	Immunology	37
Sexual Masochism	UCV-1	BEHAV-SC	Paraphilia	64
Sexual Sadism	UCV-1	BEHAV-SC	PARAPHILIA	65
Sheehan's Syndrome	UCV-1	PATHOPHYS-3	Obstetrics	66
Sheehan's Syndrome	UCV-2	OB/GYN	Obstetrics	49
Shigellosis	MC	IM-2	Infectious Disease	188
Shigellosis	UCV-1	MICRO-2	Infectious Disease	53
Shock—Hypovolemic	MC	ER	Cardiology	12
Shock—Hypovolemic	UCV-1	PATHOPHYS-1	Cardiology	24
Shock—Septic	UCV-1	MICRO-2	Infectious Disease	54
Shock—Septic	UCV-2	ER	Infectious Disease	26
Shoulder Dislocation	UCV-1	ANAT	Orthopedics	93
Shoulder Dislocation	UCV-2	SURG	Orthopedics	47
Shoulder Separation	UCV-1	ANAT	Orthopedics	94
Shy–Drager Syndrome	MC	NEURO	Neurology	262
SIADH	UCV-1	BIOCHEM	Endocrinology	30
SIADH	UCV-2	IM-1	Endocrinology	28
Sialolithiasis	UCV-1	ANAT	ENT/Ophthalmology	12
Sickle Cell Anemia	UCV-1	PATHOPHYS-2	Hematology/Oncology	36
Sickle Cell Anemia	UCV-2	PED	Hematology/Oncology	21
Sickle Cell Anemia—Vaso-occlusive Crisis	UCV-2	ER	Hematology/Oncology	23
Sideroblastic Anemia	MC	IM-1	Hematology/Oncology	129
Sigmoid Volvulus	UCV-1	ANAT	General Surgery	34
Sigmoid Volvulus	UCV-2	ER	General Surgery	20
Silicosis	UCV-1	PATHOPHYS-2	Pulmonary	93

Case Name	SER	BOOK	SubSpecialty	Case Number
Strangulated Femoral Hernia	UCV-2	SURG	General Surgery	23
Strongyloidiasis	UCV-1	MICRO-2	Infectious Disease	56
Stye	MC	ER	ENT/Ophthalmology	43
Subacute Bacterial Endocarditis	UCV-1	MICRO-1	Cardiology	5
Subacute Bacterial Endocarditis	UCV-2	IM-2	Cardiology	2
Subacute Sclerosing Panencephalitis	UCV-1	MICRO-2	Neurology	100
Subacute Sclerosing Panencephalitis	UCV-2	NEURO	Neurology	46
Subarachnoid Hemorrhage	MC	NEURO	Neurology	264
Subarachnoid Hemorrhage	UCV-1	PATHOPHYS-3	Neurology	31
Subdiaphragmatic Abscess	UCV-1	MICRO-2	Infectious Disease	57
Subdural Hematoma	UCV-1	PATHOPHYS-3	Neurology	32
Subdural Hematoma—Acute	UCV-2	ER	Neurology	35
Sublimation	UCV-1	BEHAV-SC	Defense Mechanism	25
Sudden Infant Death Syndrome (SIDS)	UCV-1	PATHOPHYS-2	Neonatology	47
Sudden Infant Death Syndrome	UCV-2	PED	Neonatology	46
Superior Vena Cava Syndrome	MC	ER	Cardiology	13
Suppurative Hidradenitis	UCV-2	SURG	Dermatology	5
Syphilis—Congenital	UCV-1	MICRO-2	Infectious Disease	58
Syphilis—Congenital	UCV-2	PED	Infectious Disease	32
Syphilis—Primary	MC	IM-2	Infectious Disease	189
Syphilis—Primary	UCV-1	MICRO-2	Infectious Disease	59
Syphilis—Secondary	UCV-1	MICRO-2	Infectious Disease	60
Syphilis—Secondary	UCV-2	IM-2	Infectious Disease	27
Syphilis—Tertiary (Aortitis)	MC	IM-2	Infectious Disease	190
Syphilis—Tertiary (Aortitis)	UCV-1	PATHOPHYS-2	Infectious Disease	45
Syphilis—Tertiary (Tabes Dorsalis)	UCV-1	MICRO-2	Infectious Disease	61
Syringomyelia	MC	NEURO	Neurology	265
Syringomyelia	UCV-1	PATHOPHYS-3	Neurology	33
Systemic Lupus Erythematosus (SLE)	UCV-1	PATHOPHYS-3	Rheumatology	95
Systemic Lupus Erythematosus (SLE)	UCV-2	IM-2	Rheumatology	56
T Takayasu's Arteritis	MC	IM-2	Rheumatology	229
Tamiflu (Oseltamivir) Therapy	UCV-1	PHARM	Infectious Disease	54
Tarasoff's Decision	UCV-2	PSYCH	Ethics	34
Tardive Dyskinesia	UCV-1	PHARM	Psychopharmacology	87
Tardive Dyskinesia	UCV-2	PSYCH	Psychopharmacology	26
Tay–Sachs Disease	UCV-1	BIOCHEM	Genetics	72
Temporal Arteritis (Giant Cell Arteritis)	UCV-1	PATHOPHYS-3	Neurology	34

Case Name	SER	BOOK	SubSpecialty	Case Number
Tic Disorder—Tourette's	UCV-1	BEHAV-SC	Child Psychiatry	40
Tic Disorder—Transient	UCV-2	PSYCH	Child	16
Tick Paralysis	UCV-1	MICRO-2	Infectious Disease	64
Tietze's Syndrome	MC	ER	Cardiology	15
Tinea Corporis (Ringworm)	MC	IM-2	Dermatology	151
Tinea Corporis (Ringworm)	UCV-1	MICRO-1	Dermatology	15
Todd's Paralysis	MC	NEURO	Neurology	266
Tonsillitis	UCV-1	ANAT	ENT/Ophthalmology	14
Torsades de Pointes	UCV-2	IM-1	Cardiology	14
Torsion of the Appendix Testis	MC	SURG	Nephrology/Urology	367
Toxemia of Pregnancy—Eclampsia	UCV-2	OB/GYN	Obstetrics	51
Toxemia of Pregnancy—Preeclampsia	UCV-1	PATHOPHYS-3	Obstetrics	67
Toxic Epidermal Necrolysis	MC	ER	Dermatology	20
Toxic Megacolon	MC	SURG	Gastroenterology	342
Toxic Megacolon	UCV-1	PATHOPHYS-1	Gastroenterology	101
Toxic Shock Syndrome (TSS)	UCV-1	MICRO-2	Gynecology	106
Toxic Shock Syndrome (TSS)	UCV-2	OB/GYN	Gynecology	27
Toxoplasmosis	MC	IM-2	Infectious Disease	191
Toxoplasmosis	UCV-1	MICRO-2	Infectious Disease	65
Toxoplasmosis—Congenital	UCV-2	PED	Infectious Disease	34
Tracheoesophageal Fistula	MC	PED	Gastroenterology	313
Tracheoesophageal Fistula	UCV-1	ANAT	Gastroenterology	23
Transfusion Reaction—Acute Hemolytic	UCV-1	PATHOPHYS-2	Hematology/Oncology	39
Transfusion Reaction—Febrile Nonhemolytic	UCV-1	PATHOPHYS-2	Hematology/Oncology	40
Transfusion Reaction—Hemolytic	MC	ER	Hematology/Oncology	56
Transient Ischemic Attack	UCV-2	ER	Neurology	36
Traveler's Diarrhea	UCV-1	MICRO-1	Gastroenterology	40
Trichinosis	MC	IM-2	Infectious Disease	192
Trichinosis	UCV-1	MICRO-2	Infectious Disease	66
Tricyclic Antidepressant Overdose	UCV-1	PHARM	Psychopharmacology	89
Tricyclic Antidepressant Overdose	UCV-2	ER	Psychopharmacology	42
Trigeminal Neuralgia	UCV-1	ANAT	Neurology	72
Trigeminal Neuralgia	UCV-2	NEURO	Neurology	49
Tuberculosis—Miliary	UCV-1	MICRO-2	Infectious Disease	67
Tuberculosis—Pulmonary	UCV-1	MICRO-2	Infectious Disease	68
Tuberculosis—Pulmonary	UCV-2	IM-2	Infectious Disease	29
Tubo-Ovarian Abscess	MC	OB/GYN	Gynecology	284
Tubulointerstitial Disease—Drug-Induced	UCV-1	PHARM	Nephrology/Urology	60

Case Name	SER	BOOK	SubSpecialty	Case Number
Tularemia	MC	IM-2	Infectious Disease	193
Tularemia	UCV-1	MICRO-2	Infectious Disease	69
Twin Pregnancy	UCV-2	OB/GYN	Obstetrics	52
Typhoid Fever	UCV-1	MICRO-2	Infectious Disease	70
Typhoid Fever	UCV-2	IM-2	Infectious Disease	30
Ulcerative Colitis	UCV-1	PATHOPHYS-1	Gastroenterology	102
Ulcerative Colitis	UCV-2	IM-1	Gastroenterology	40
Umbilical Hernia	MC	SURG	General Surgery	363
Urate Nephropathy	UCV-1	PATHOPHYS-2	Nephrology/Urology	72
Ureteral Injury—Iatrogenic	UCV-1	ANAT	General Surgery	37
Urethritis	UCV-2	ER	Infectious Disease	27
Urethritis—Nongonococcal	UCV-1	MICRO-2	Infectious Disease	71
Urinary Tract Infection (UTI)	UCV-1	MICRO-2	Infectious Disease	72
Urinary Tract Infection (UTI)	UCV-2	IM-2	Infectious Disease	31
Urticaria	MC	ER	Dermatology	21
Urticaria	UCV-1	MICRO-1	Dermatology	16
Uterine Fibroids	UCV-1	PATHOPHYS-3	OB/GYN Gynecology	58
Uterine Fibroids	UCV-2	OB/GYN	Gynecology	28
Uterine Leiomyosarcoma	UCV-1	PATHOPHYS-3	Gynecology	59
Uterine Prolapse with Cystocele	UCV-1	ANAT	Gynecology	40
Uterine Prolapse with Cystocele	UCV-2	OB/GYN	Gynecology	29
UTI with Staphylococcus saprophyticus	UCV-1	MICRO-2	Infectious Disease	73
Uveitis	MC	ER	ENT/Ophthalmology	37
Uveitis	UCV-1	PATHOPHYS-1	ENT/Ophthalmology	74
Vaginismus	UCV-1	BEHAV-SC	Somatoform Disorders	95
Vaginitis—Atrophic	MC	OB/GYN	Gynecology	285
Vaginitis—Candidal	UCV-2	OB/GYN	Gynecology	30
Vaginitis—Trichomonas	UCV-2	OB/GYN	Gynecology	31
Varicella Zoster (Chickenpox)	UCV-1	MICRO-2	Infectious Disease	74
Varicella Zoster (Chickenpox)	UCV-2	PED	Infectious Disease	35
Varicose Veins	MC	SURG	General Surgery	364
Varicose Veins	UCV-1	ANAT	General Surgery	38
Vasectomy	UCV-1	ANAT	Nephrology/Urology	48
Ventricular Fibrillation	UCV-2	ER	Cardiology	6
Ventricular Flutter	MC	ER	Cardiology	16
Ventricular Septal Defect	UCV-1	ANAT	Cardiology	8
Ventricular Septal Defect	UCV-2	PED	Cardiology	3
Verapamil Side Effects	UCV-1	PHARM	Cardiology	11

W

	Case Name	SER	BOOK	SubSpecialty	Case Number
	Whipple's Disease	UCV-1	MICRO-1	Gastroenterology	43
	Whooping Cough	MC	PED	Infectious Disease	327
	Whooping Cough	UCV-1	MICRO-2	Infectious Disease	76
	Wilms' Tumor	UCV-1	PATHOPHYS-2	Nephrology/Urology	73
	Wilms' Tumor	UCV-2	PED	Nephrology/Urology	48
	Wilson's Disease	UCV-1	BIOCHEM	Gastroenterology	41
	Wilson's Disease	UCV-2	PED	Gastroenterology	9
	Wiskott–Aldrich Syndrome	UCV-1	PATHOPHYS-2	Hematology/Oncology	43
	Wiskott–Aldrich Syndrome	UCV-2	PED	Hematology/Oncology	23
	Withholding Treatment	UCV-2	PSYCH	Ethics	35
	Wolff–Parkinson–White Syndrome	UCV-1	PATHOPHYS-1	Cardiology	28
	Wolff–Parkinson–White Syndrome	UCV-2	IM-1	Cardiology	15
	Wrist—Barton's Fracture	MC	SURG	Orthopedics	378
	Wrist—Carpal Tunnel Syndrome	UCV-1	ANAT	Orthopedics	98
	Wrist—Colles' Fracture	UCV-2	SURG	Orthopedics	49
	Wrist—Scaphoid Fracture	MC	SURG	Orthopedics	379
	Wrist—Scaphoid Fracture	UCV-1	ANAT	Orthopedics	99
	Wrist Slash Injury	UCV-1	ANAT	Orthopedics	100
X	Xeroderma Pigmentosum	UCV-1	BIOCHEM	Genetics	74
	X-Linked Hypogammaglobulinemia	UCV-1	MICRO-2	Immunology	6
Y	Yaws	UCV-1	MICRO-2	Infectious Disease	77
	Yellow Fever	UCV-1	MICRO-2	Infectious Disease	78
	Yersinia Enterocolitis	UCV-1	MICRO-1	Gastroenterology	44
Z	Zidovudine Toxicity	UCV-1	PHARM	Infectious Disease	56
	Zollinger–Ellison Syndrome	MC	IM-1	Gastroenterology	112
	Zollinger–Ellison Syndrome	UCV-1	PATHOPHYS-1	Gastroenterology	103